No Patient Left Behind:

A Comprehensive Guide to Inclusive Clinical Research

Ana Macedo

No Patient Left Behind: A Comprehensive Guide to Inclusive Clinical Research

Ana Macedo

1st Edition, May 2024

Copyright © AMM 2024

All rights reserved. No part of this book may be reproduced, distributed, or transmitted in any form or by any means, including photocopying, recording, or other electronic or mechanical methods, without the prior written permission of the author, except in the case of brief quotations embodied in critical reviews and certain other noncommercial uses permitted by copyright law.

Published by AMM

This book is dedicated to all the people with whom, over more than 20 years, I have crossed paths in multiple clinical research projects, and also to those who are just starting out and have the opportunity to do excellent clinical research, which is necessarily inclusive clinical research.

Table of Contents

SECTION 1 - WHY TALK ABOUT INCLUSIVE RESEARCH? 7

CHAPTER 1 - INCLUSIVE CLINICAL RESEARCH 9
CHAPTER 2 - INCLUSIVE LANGUAGE 15

SECTION II - WHAT IS MEANT BY CLINICAL STUDY? 23

CHAPTER 3 - CLINICAL STUDY: GENERAL CONCEPTS 25
CHAPTER 4 - CLASSIFICATION OF CLINICAL STUDIES......................... 29
CHAPTER 5 - DEVELOPMENT OF NEW DRUGS 37
CHAPTER 6 - REAL-WORLD EVIDENCE... 41

SECTION III - HOW TO DESIGN A CLINICAL STUDY 45

CHAPTER 7 - PROTOCOL STRUCTURE 47
CHAPTER 8 - RESEARCH QUESTION 61
CHAPTER 9 - OBJECTIVES AND ENDPOINTS 69
CHAPTER 10 - STUDY DESIGNS 75
CHAPTER 11 - POPULATION 81
CHAPTER 12 - METHODOLOGY AND PROCEDURES 85
CHAPTER 13 - ETHICAL AND REGULATORY FRAMEWORK 93
CHAPTER 14 - INFORMATION FOR THE PARTICIPANT AND INFORMED CONSENT 97

SECTION IV - INTERVENTION STUDIES................................... 101

CHAPTER 15 - CLINICAL TRIAL - CONCEPT.. 103
CHAPTER 16 - PHASES OF CLINICAL TRIALS 107
CHAPTER 17 - PHASE 1 CLINICAL TRIALS 109
CHAPTER 18 - PHASE 2 CLINICAL TRIALS 119
CHAPTER 19 - PHASE 3 CLINICAL TRIALS 129
CHAPTER 20 - PHASE 4 CLINICAL TRIALS 143
CHAPTER 21 - OTHER INTERVENTION STUDIES 147

SECTION V - OBSERVATIONAL STUDIES REAL-WORLD DATA 155

CHAPTER 22 - OBSERVATIONAL STUDIES - CONCEPT 157
CHAPTER 23 - CROSS-SECTIONAL STUDIES 159
CHAPTER 24 - COHORT STUDIES 163
CHAPTER 25 - CASE-CONTROL STUDIES 169

SECTION VI - DATA COLLECTION 175

CHAPTER 26 - DATA COLLECTION 177
CHAPTER 27 - INCLUSIVE LANGUAGE IN DATA COLLECTION INSTRUMENTS 185

SECTION VII - DATA AND RESULTS 191

CHAPTER 28 - VARIABLES 193
CHAPTER 29 - STATISTICAL ANALYSIS - GENERAL ASPECTS 197
CHAPTER 30 - STATISTICAL ANALYSIS - DESCRIPTIVE ANALYSES.... 205
CHAPTER 31 - STATISTICAL ANALYSIS – COMPARISONS AND ASSOCIATIONS 209
CHAPTER 32 - SAMPLE SIZE AND SAMPLE CHARACTERISTICS 219

BIBLIOGRAPHY 227

ABOUT THE AUTHOR 237

Section 1 - Why Talk About Inclusive Research?

Chapter 1 - Inclusive Clinical Research

Why do we need to talk about inclusive clinical research?

Mainly because we are aware that clinical research has left out many people, claiming scientific criteria that are not always plausible or true. Do you feel confident using a certain medication in an 80-year-old woman, knowing that its pharmacokinetic characteristics were determined in men under 30 years old, and its efficacy and safety profiles were defined for people without other pathologies, who were not taking any other medications, and who were under 65 years old? Maybe you have never thought about it, but one thing is certain: everyone needs medication at some point in their lives, and, in general, older people need it more than younger ones.

The arguments for excluding people belonging to minority groups or those with comorbidities or using multiple medications from clinical studies are varied and include reasons such as the heterogeneity arising from these factors and the decrease in the internal validity of the studies. Both are correct arguments, but what about our ethical commitment? And the external validity of the studies?

Talking about inclusive research is much more than talking about the inclusion of all people in clinical studies; it's talking about the objectives of those studies, the language we use when writing our protocols or questionnaires, and the teams that design and implement the studies.

The clinical research you should aspire to must necessarily consider people in all their diversity, including their biological, environmental, social, and behavioral characteristics, ultimately reflecting the World Health Organization's (WHO) definition of health and its principles (1), which establish, among others, that:

"Health is a state of complete physical, mental, and social well-being and not merely the absence of disease or infirmity."

"The enjoyment of the highest attainable standard of health is one of the fundamental rights of every human being without distinction of race, religion, political belief, economic or social condition."

I go further because, when rereading these definitions, I had the feeling that they no longer translate what I consider to be true inclusion. If I could propose changes, I would suggest not using the word "race," but instead physiognomic characteristics, ancestry, and geographic origin, and, on the other hand, I would add (without distinction of) sex, gender identity, or sexual orientation.

Despite the principles outlined above, clinical research has left out many people. Women, people belonging to sexual and gender minorities, pregnant women, older people, people from different sociocultural backgrounds, obese people, and people with non-white skin are some examples of individuals and groups that have been systematically excluded, undermining their right to health equity.

In a 2020 publication (2), 32,000 individuals who participated in clinical trials of new drugs in the United States (US) were analyzed. Of the people included, only 8% were African American, and only 30% were 65 years or older. According to the US Census, 14.4% of the population was African American (3). The situation is all the more serious when we know that, on the one hand, these groups are underrepresented in clinical studies, and on the other hand, they have specificities and increased prevalence of certain diseases, resulting from both genetic factors and the socioeconomic and cultural context. Therefore, we run the risk that the people who would benefit most from the results of certain clinical studies are not included in them. This results not only in an asymmetry and inequality in early access to a potential new treatment but also makes it impossible for drugs to be optimized according to the characteristics of these individuals, with respect to, for example, doses, frequencies of administration, or safety profile.

You may be thinking that there are clinical or even ethical reasons for this to happen. For example, women were systematically excluded from participation in phase 1 clinical trials. Why? Because it was assumed that there could always be a risk of pregnancy and, as such, the risk of exposure to an experimental drug in its initial phase of study was not justified. The same was assumed for not including older people, and by older, you can understand over 40 or 50 years old, people with a higher risk of disease, or those who were taking other medications. What is the practical result of these choices? The pharmacokinetics and pharmacodynamics of most drugs marketed today were studied in young (and white) men.

As for obese people, people from different sociocultural backgrounds, or people from sexual and gender minorities, the "official" reasons for their non-inclusion in many clinical studies relate to maximizing the internal validity of the results. It is true that heterogeneity reduces the validity of the study, but this is not a sufficient reason for many of the choices made, especially because we have to assume that the type of selection that has been made has a huge impact on the external validity of those same results.

As an example, I would like you to reflect on the validity of the results of most clinical trials regarding women, black, elderly, and obese people, or transgender people, who will take medications assuming a pharmacokinetic profile, efficacy, and safety determined in clinical trials in which they did not participate.

Aware of this reality, several institutions have spoken out in favor of more inclusive clinical research (4-7).

The WHO has published guidelines on promoting the inclusion of women, children, and other underrepresented populations in clinical trials. These guidelines emphasize the importance of involving these populations in all phases of the research process, from study design to data analysis and dissemination of results.

I would like to introduce a brief note here, drawing your attention to a slightly different but equally relevant topic: how are the teams that design and decide on the type of clinical studies to be conducted constituted?

So far, we have talked about the inclusion of study participants and the importance of their representativeness, covering the spectrum of human diversity. I would like you to also think about the issue of political, scientific, and business decisions in the field of health, and consequently, clinical research. It is essential, as the WHO recommendation underlines, to involve different types of people in a representative and inclusive way in the decision-making, design, planning, and analysis of clinical studies.

In 2020, the FDA published a document titled "Enhancing the Diversity of Clinical Trial Populations — Eligibility Criteria, Enrollment Practices, and Trial Designs Guidance for Industry" (8), showing not only its concern with the underrepresentation of some population groups but also the need to promote immediate action by sponsoring entities, namely the pharmaceutical industry. The document explicitly mentions the need to consider both the demographic characteristics of the study populations (e.g., sex, physiognomic characteristics, geographic origin, age, place of residence) and the non-demographic characteristics of the populations (e.g., patients with single or multiple organ failure, comorbidities, people with disabilities, individuals with obesity or extreme thinness, and populations with low-prevalence diseases or conditions). The document safeguards situations in which certain individuals or population groups should not be included in a particular clinical trial for safety reasons, reflecting on situations in which the reasons for non-inclusion are justified.

In addition to this document, the FDA previously published another aimed at promoting the inclusion of people of different "races" and ethnicities (9), adolescents (10), and children (11).

From the various documents and recommendations, there is a need to collect sufficient information to allow for the analysis of minority groups, which translates into having a sufficient number of people in study samples, but also into planning the collection of the necessary information for their characterization.

In general, public institutions, companies, and research teams seem to agree on the importance of making clinical research inclusive to ensure that healthcare interventions are effective and safe for all individuals, regardless of their origin or identity. But for this to become a reality, each of us needs to do our part in every clinical research project.

To conclude this chapter, I propose a challenge. When you think of a clinical research project, ask yourself if that project is sufficiently inclusive. Divide your analysis into four parts:

1. Theme and objectives: Do the theme and objectives of your project take diversity and inclusion into account? Are sufficiently explicit and targeted questions asked to analyze data from minority groups, increasing health knowledge about them?

2. Study participants: Who are the people being studied, and why were certain individuals included or excluded?

3. Language: Is the language used in study materials, including protocol, informed consent, participant information sheet, and data collection materials, neutral and inclusive?

4. Research team: Does the project design and conception include people representative of different groups, particularly underrepresented groups? Is the analysis and interpretation of results shared by a group of people that reflects this same diversity?

Chapter 2 - Inclusive Language

Before delving into methodological topics such as the definition and classification of clinical studies, and since this manual is about inclusive clinical research, I chose to first address aspects related to people. I don't claim to be able to include all those who have been systematically discriminated against. When you think about discrimination in this context, I would like you to consider that it can happen in different ways, as we saw at the end of the previous chapter, and I'll remind you again here. Discrimination is, for example:

- The fact that people from certain groups are explicitly excluded from clinical studies, or, despite not being explicitly excluded, in practice they end up not being included (the eligibility criteria don't state they can't participate, but by the end of the study they are not included).

- The study objectives do not consider the analysis of minority or vulnerable population subgroups.

- The way questions are worded, conditioning responses into categories that are not always inclusive.

- The language used in all materials, from the study protocol to the informed consent or study questionnaires.

It's important to consider that some people have been systematically discriminated against in the context of clinical research, but also how we can effectively make our studies more inclusive.

Over the next few pages, we will focus on language. One of the main sources of discrimination and non-inclusion is precisely communication and language, which creates barriers and lack of trust. It's critical that we make the effort, because it still is an effort, to use neutral terms and avoid words that may have pejorative connotations (12).

I know many people complain about the difficulty of using gender-neutral language, for example: "We always have to say 'they' and 'them'" (and still, we're not including non-binary gender identities). I agree, it's not simple, much less fluid, especially in Romance languages where most words have an assigned gender (feminine or masculine). But, despite not being simple, it's important.

Language neutrality allows reducing stereotypes and what we call unconscious bias, i.e., assumptions that our brain makes a priori without being aware of it, but which lead to discrimination.

To give you some everyday examples, by saying "the doctor" when referring to all people who practice the profession, we are conditioning our mental image to be a man in a white coat with a stethoscope. If you ask young children to draw doctors or astronauts they will probably draw men, while if we ask them to think of nurses they will probably depict women. Is this related to the number of professionals in each field? To what we are exposed to in the media? Of course, but it is reinforced by the terminology we use.

Another important and complex aspect of using neutral language is to allow no one to feel discriminated against when reading (or listening to) a particular text, in this case, clinical study materials, whether the protocol, questionnaires, or presentation of results.

If in oral language this can be such a complex exercise that it impedes or disrupts communication, I believe that in written language it is not only possible but also extraordinarily useful.

I don't intend to be exhaustive on this matter, and I apologize in advance if throughout this book I was unable to use language as neutral as I would like; please believe it was not for lack of effort or willingness. To conclude this point, I would like to leave some practical suggestions regarding common words and expressions in the context of clinical research:

- Try to avoid terms like "the patients" or "the sick", replacing them with "people who are ill" or "people with the disease...", or even "individuals with ...".

- Similarly, try to avoid using "the doctor" or "the researcher". If possible, replace with "the medical team" or "the research team". If it is not a team at all, but a single person, you can use "healthcare professional" or "research professional".

- Carefully assess whether the words you are using are nouns or adjectives/attributes. For example, we don't say "the diabetic" or "the hypertensive", but rather "the person with diabetes" or "the person with hypertension". In the same way that we don't say "the transgender", but rather "the transgender person". In either context, we simultaneously seek two things: first to use gender-neutral language, and then, to assume that the person is not defined by the disease or their gender identity, but that these are attributes, so they should be used as adjectives.

Throughout this book we will talk about minority groups and groups considered vulnerable or underrepresented, to such an extent that it jeopardizes their right to health equity. In other words, and as we have seen before, the fact that there are people who are systematically excluded from clinical studies conditions that their health outcomes are worse, with a direct influence on their quality of life and average life expectancy.

Before moving on, let's define some terms and concepts that I will use over the next pages. The definitions I propose are not intended to establish a language glossary, but only to create a referential that allows us to have the same understanding of the terms used.

Sex and gender

Sex (sex assigned at birth) is classified as female, male or intersex (the designation intersex applies to people whose sexual characteristics, including chromosomes or anatomy of sexual and/or reproductive organs, are not typical of female or male sex, being a very rare condition). Sex assigned at birth is defined by the biological and physiological characteristics, such as the anatomy, reproductive and sexual organs, chromosomes and hormonal environment of each individual (13).

Gender is a social construct of behaviors, attitudes, expressions and roles. Gender identity is how the person identifies themselves in relation to this social construct and can be binary - feminine and masculine - or non-binary, in the sense that the person identifies neither with feminine nor masculine. In this way, we can assume that there is a gender spectrum that varies between feminine and masculine, and may have an infinity of intermediate points (13).

The concept of gender is operationalized in individual terms as "gender identity" and "gender expression", which refers to how the person presents themselves to society with respect to established gender patterns.

It is also important to clarify what is meant by cisgender and transgender person. The term cisgender means that the gender the person identifies with matches the sex assigned to them at birth. Conversely, the term transgender means that the gender the person identifies with does not match the sex assigned to them at birth.

Later on we will talk about ways of asking and classifying gender identity in the context of clinical studies, so I choose not to address the issue here.

Physiognomic aspects and ancestry

Perhaps the title you were expecting for what I will address in this subchapter was "race and ethnicity", however, in biological and genetic terms it does not make sense to speak of several races with regard to human beings.

The concept of "race" as we use it on a daily basis is relatively recent in human history and derives from the social construction of racism. A document on "Race and Racism", published in 2019 by the American Association of Biological Anthropologists (14), says:

> «Race does not provide an accurate representation of human biological variation. It never has and never will. There has not been and is not a biological basis for racial categories. Humans are not divided biologically into distinct continental types or racial genetic clusters. Instead, the Western concept of race must be understood as a classification system that emerged from and in support of European colonialism, oppression, and discrimination. It thus does not have its roots in biological reality, but in policies of discrimination. Because of this, over the last five centuries, race has become a social reality that structures societies and how we experience the world. In this regard, race is real, as is racism, and both have real biological consequences.
>
> Humans share the vast majority (99.9%) of our DNA in common. Individuals nevertheless exhibit substantial genetic and phenotypic variability. Genome/environment interactions, local and regional biological changes through time, and genetic exchange among populations have produced the biological diversity we see in

humans today. Such genetic variability is not distributed across our species in a manner that maps clearly onto socially-recognized racial groups. This is true even for aspects of human variation that we frequently emphasize in discussions of race, such as facial features, skin color and hair type. No group of people is, or ever has been, biologically homogeneous or "pure." These categories of "race" are not scientifically valid, and do not provide an accurate picture of human biological diversity. This does not mean that "race" does not exist or that racism is not real; race exists because racism exists, and racism has biological consequences. (...)

(...) Because racial categories do not represent biological subdivisions of humanity, we should not expect races to be identifiable by characteristic allele frequencies or specific genetic variants. Human biological variation is real, of course, and can sometimes cluster on the basis of geography, which may roughly map onto some notions of race. The existence of these genetic clusters, however, does not support a genetic basis for traditional racial categories (based largely on continental ancestry), much less a biological basis for the discrimination that racial categories have been used to justify.»

Taking into account what we just read, it doesn't make sense to talk about "race" from a biological point of view, but the term continues to be used to define population groups with specific physiognomic and genetic characteristics. It is crucial, in the context of clinical research, to understand what characteristics we are talking about and what is the best way to designate them when asking a question in a questionnaire or establishing an analysis objective in a study protocol. Is it the geographic origin that we want to know? Ancestry? Skin color? Sociocultural context? Then, that should be our question.

For lack of a better alternative, I chose to use the word "race" in quotation marks throughout the text, understanding it as expressed above.

Ethnicity is not another way of saying "race", they are not synonyms, nor does it translate the aspects mentioned above such as geographic origin, ancestry, skin color or sociocultural context. Ethnicity refers to a group of people who mutually identify as being part of the same culture, history, language, society or nation. Thus, ethnicity is a sociocultural and self-classification concept, it is a person's own identity, and should not be inferred by other people based only on the surrounding context. Again, if asked in the context of a clinical study, we must know exactly what we intend to find out, and frame our question accordingly.

Section II - What is meant by clinical study?

Chapter 3 - Clinical Study: General Concepts

I am often asked what a clinical study is. Although we can deviate a little from the definition and make our own assumptions, the Good Clinical Practice Guidelines define what we can call a "clinical study"(15).

"Clinical trial or study" means any systematic research conducted on human beings or based on individual health data, designed to discover or verify the distribution or effect of health factors, health states or outcomes, health or disease processes, effect and safety of health interventions or services, through biological, behavioral, social or organizational aspects."

I now propose that you take a closer look at this definition, trying to identify the key aspects that allow us to designate a research project as a clinical study.

Let's try to break down the definition and, to begin with, let's establish some basic rules:

- A clinical study must be a systematic study, what does this mean?

It means that the study is conducted according to the scientific method or, more pragmatically, that the different components of this study are planned and defined in advance, from the research question to the objectives, procedures, population included and how to analyze the data, usually documented in a study protocol (see Chapter 7).

- A clinical study is, by definition, conducted on human beings and evaluates individual health data.

This means that a clinical study evaluates health data from several individuals, each of whom constitutes a unit of analysis, that is, there is a database per individual. If we have a study in which we analyze, for example, aggregated health data from several countries, this study, according to current legislation, should not be called a clinical study, because the data, although being health data and referring to individuals, are not being analyzed individually.

- Thirdly, the purpose of the study must be considered. We can only qualify a study as a clinical trial if its objective is to verify the distribution or effect of health factors, health states or outcomes, health or disease processes, efficacy and safety of health interventions or services, through biological, behavioral, social or organizational aspects.

This component of the definition of clinical trial is broad and includes studies as diverse as those that address the biological or epidemiological mechanism of a disease, the effect of a drug or the functioning of a health organization.

In summary, a clinical study is a systematic scientific study that assesses the health or disease status of individuals, but also of health services, and may include biological, behavioral, social or organizational aspects. A clinical trial is a subtype of clinical study in which an experimental drug is evaluated, but there are many clinical studies that are not clinical trials, as we will see below.

Chapter 4 - Classification of Clinical Studies

Taking into account the definition of a clinical study that we saw in the previous chapter, I think you have no doubt that, in the global context of clinical research, there are several types of studies. The classification and designation of each of them can be done in different ways, that is, a study can be classified according to its objectives, population, time, use of previous data or data to be collected later, or according to its specific methodological design. In my opinion, none of these classifications are perfect, as they do not cover all the characteristics that make a study unique, as there are always particularities that have not been taken into account, but they are useful for organizing them.

Before trying to systematize clinical studies from these multiple elements, I challenge you to think in a binary way about some characteristics:

1. Interventional study versus observational study: We classify a study as experimental if interventions are planned, pharmacological or not, that are not part of routine clinical practice. We classify a study as observational if the study involves only the observation and recording of what is routinely done, without modifying clinical practice (Figure 1).

Figure 1 - Interventional study versus observational study.

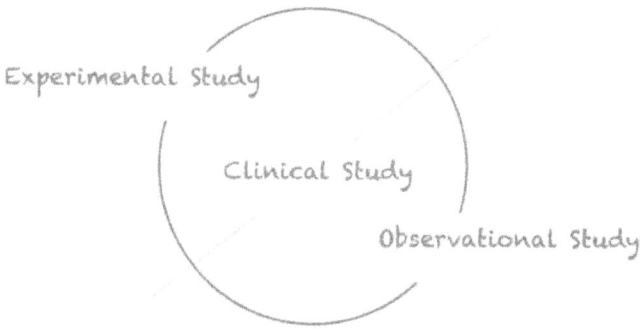

2. Clinical/therapeutic study versus epidemiological study: we classify the study according to the research question and the type of objective being analyzed. Studies of a clinical or therapeutic nature focus, for example, on assessing the effect of a particular drug or clinical intervention, while studies of an epidemiological nature focus, for example, on the incidence or prevalence of a disease, assessing risk factors or prognostic factors.

3. Clinical/therapeutic studies and epidemiological studies can be interventional or observational (Figure 2).

4. Disease-based study versus community-based study: we classify the study according to the characteristics of the population to be evaluated. When the study is carried out in the community, we assume that it will include both healthy people and people with some kind of disease, but this is not a factor that influences their inclusion in the study.

Figure 2 - Interventional study versus observational study - epidemiological versus clinical/therapeutic nature.

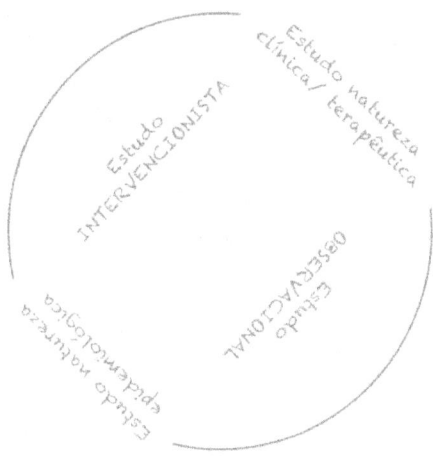

4. Longitudinal study versus cross-sectional study: we classify the study in terms of "time", in the sense that we define whether the study evaluates a single point in time, "snapshot type", or if there is a follow-up of the people included, "movie type". Longitudinal studies can be subclassified as retrospective (data refer to the past, compared to the start of the study) or prospective (data are collected in the present and future, compared to the start of the study).

5. Primary versus secondary data source study: strictly speaking, we should not consider secondary data source studies as "true" clinical studies (see previous chapter), as these studies do not analyze each person individually, but rather an analysis of aggregated data already collected in previous studies.

Figure 3 - Classification of studies in the context of clinical research.

Clinical and epidemiological research						
Research using primary data sources				Research using secondary data sources		
Interventional studies		Observational studies				
Clinical	Epidemiological	Clinical	Epidemiological	Ecological	Reviews	Meta-analysis
• Clinical trials • Other interventional studies	• Prevention (with intervention)	• Drugs • Diagnosis • Prognosis	• Disease distribution • Disease causes • Risk and prevention	• Aggregated data	• Narrative reviews • Systematic reviews	• Drugs • Diagnosis • Disease distribution

Although the classifications are not perfect, for practical purposes it is important to be able to classify the type of study that one wants to do or that one is analyzing, as the most appropriate type of methodology and the applicable ethical and legal principles and requirements will directly depend on it. A classification proposal that includes the most common studies in the context of clinical research is presented in Figure 3.

A final observation just to mention that studies in biological models, genetic and molecular studies, or studies in animal models are not considered clinical studies, since, by definition, clinical studies analyze human beings.

I now propose a more detailed examination and some practical examples of the presented classification, evaluating its multiple factors.

Let's recall the definition from the previous chapter: Clinical studies are systematic studies in human beings in which health data are evaluated individually. They can be divided according to:

- objectives

- included population

- type of design/methodology

To classify a study according to the type of objectives, it is necessary to take into account whether the study aims to describe a situation, compare groups or associate variables, but also the specific situation to be analyzed. For example, you may have a study that wants to evaluate the effect of a new drug by comparing it with an existing drug, or a study that aims to describe the characteristics of people with a certain pathology, or a study that aims to determine which factors have a good prognosis after a certain diagnosis. If the focus is on the population, there may be studies carried out on healthy people or on patients with certain demographic characteristics, and studies carried out in the community, in primary care or in a hospital setting.

When thinking about study design, studies can be classified according to their time perspective: cross-sectional or longitudinal and, in the latter case, retrospective or prospective, while also being classified according to their epidemiological or clinical, observational or interventionist nature.

In epidemiological studies, that is, studies that aim to evaluate aspects related to the distribution, causes, risk and prevention of a disease in a given population or community, the most common designs are cohort studies, case-control studies and cross-sectional studies. Examples of each of these designs include

- Assessment of risk factors for major cardiovascular events in the LGBTQ+ population residing in the state of New York - Cohort study.

- Determination of the association between the use of drug X and the occurrence of acute liver failure - Case-control study.

- Assessment of the prevalence of psoriasis in people aged between 18 and 25 years old - Cross-sectional study.

Clinical studies have different objectives, such as assessing the efficacy and safety of new drugs or interventions, whether therapeutic or diagnostic (interventional studies), assessing the efficacy and safety of drugs and procedures commonly used in routine clinical practice (observational studies), assessing prognostic factors of a disease or assessing the reliability of complementary diagnostic means.

Examples include:

- Evaluation of the efficacy and safety of a new drug, still under development, for the treatment of postpartum depression compared to an alternative already available on the market - Interventional study.

• Comparison between two drugs already marketed with indication for use in the prevention of migraine attacks, in the context of routine clinical practice - Observational study.

• Comparison between a new complementary diagnostic tool and a technique commonly used in clinical practice for the detection of gallstones in obese people - Interventional study.

• Study to evaluate factors of good prognosis in people over 75 years of age with septic shock admitted to intensive care - Observational study.

Chapter 5 - Development of New Drugs

Although this manual does not specifically deal with the process of research and development of new drugs, I believe it is important to provide an overview of the subject, especially if you are not familiar with the process, as clinical studies, particularly clinical trials, are an essential part of this process and are vital for new drugs to be approved and marketed.

The process of research and development of new drugs begins long before clinical studies. Depending on the drug and its potential use, action models are developed, and mechanisms of action are tested in vitro or in digital and virtual models, which may lead to the identification of one or more components that could be developed into a drug. This leads to chemical or biological synthesis that enables the compound to exist and be used in new experimental models. These models can be, for example, cell or animal models. Only after demonstrating safety and activity in animal models can a potential new drug be tested in humans.

The research of a new drug in humans occurs with the development and conduction of so-called Phase 1 clinical studies. The different phases of clinical studies are described later in this book, so I will not go into detail here. If the results of Phase 1 studies are positive, meaning the compound is shown to be safe and has a good pharmacokinetic and pharmacodynamic profile, the research process continues, and Phase 2 studies are initiated. Again, if the results of Phase 2 are positive, the process moves on to Phase 3. Only at the end of Phase 3, and after more than one positive Phase 3 study, can the entity that is developing the new drug and intends to market it apply to the competent authorities to review the process, and if they have a favorable opinion, they will issue the Marketing Authorization, which will allow the new drug to be made available and marketed.

In the process of developing a new drug, thousands of potential compounds are initiated, of which two or three reach the human research phase, and the process is often interrupted before that happens, either for safety reasons or because the mechanism of action is not consistent. Of the few compounds that reach Phase 1 testing, an even smaller number obtain positive results that allow them to reach Phases 2 and 3, and it is easy to deduce that those that actually reach the market are a minimal proportion.

If we think about the financial and human effort involved in the different phases, we will realize that it is a complex, time-consuming, and very expensive process. On average, it is estimated that more than 10 years (and many millions of dollars spent) are needed from the pre-clinical phase until it is possible to obtain a marketing authorization.

Of course, there are situations where the process can be "accelerated", as was the case with vaccine and treatment tests in the context of COVID-19, but these situations are very specific and need to be properly justified, as they require a huge effort from all parties involved and may involve risks due to the reduced exposure and observation time of the potential new drug.

After a drug is approved and marketed, the clinical research process continues. Phase 4 clinical studies and observational studies (also known as real-world studies) begin, which will allow the evaluation of the drug's effects and safety in much larger population groups, over a longer period of time, and under real-world conditions.

Eventually, other types of studies will be possible, such as systematic reviews and meta-analyses, which will allow the aggregation of data from clinical trials and observational studies, or economic evaluation studies, which will allow the assessment of the cost-benefit ratio of the new drug, the latter being essential for the reimbursement application processes that may occur after the marketing authorization of a drug.

The following figure summarizes the main characteristics of Phase 1 to 4 clinical research. In the description of Phase 2 clinical studies, the term surrogate endpoints appears, i.e., these are endpoints that indirectly assess the situations or diseases to be evaluated; an example of this is the determination of PSA (Prostate Specific Antigen) to assess the evolution or therapeutic response in prostate cancer.

Figure 4 - Phases of clinical research.

	Clinical Trials			
	Phase 1	Phase 2	Phase 3	Phase 4
Methodology	Open, non-controlled studies	Comparative, randomized and blinded studies or open non-comparative studies Surrogate endpoints	Comparative, randomized, double-blind trials	Post-marketing Observational studies or randomized trials
Participants	Healthy volunteers	Patients	Patients	Patients
Number of people	Few	Medium	High	Very high
Objectives	Pharmacokinetics Pharmacodynamics Safety	Safety Doses Efficacy	Efficacy Safety	Effectiveness Long-term safety Interactions
Duration	Short	Short/medium	Medium/long	Very long

Chapter 6 - Real-World Evidence

The term Real-World Evidence has been gradually introduced into our daily lives, translating into data derived from information obtained in observational clinical studies, i.e., studies conducted in a real-life context (16). This type of information is different from that obtained in an experimental setting, such as in clinical studies (17).

We can obtain health data in a real-world context from observational clinical or epidemiological studies, which evaluate previously defined objectives and, as in the case of clinical studies, have a protocol that explains in detail the population that can participate, the methodology used, including how the data will be collected and analyzed, and the processes that will be carried out during the study. Unlike clinical trials, observational studies do not involve any intervention in the participants.

In addition to observational studies, real-world health data can come from national registries, specific registries promoted by study groups or patient organizations, which regularly collect and store information on a particular health and/or disease topic.

It is important to keep in mind that, as in any clinical study, experimental or observational, a registry requires prior consent from participants and approval from the corresponding ethics committee, which depends on the type and purpose of the registry.

Real-world health data, especially that obtained in the context of observational studies (whose methodology I will describe in detail below), are particularly useful as they reflect reality with all its complications and adversities.

Observational studies are conducted in two different types of situations: situations where the study objective does not allow the use of an experimental design, for example, all studies that refer to the incidence, prevalence, lethality, characterization of the type of patients, transmission or mechanisms of a disease; and situations where we want to evaluate the effects of a drug or other intervention, but we want to do it as close as possible to real conditions. Always within this issue of drug evaluation, we have certain study objectives, such as evaluating adherence to a particular therapy, which can only be determined in observational studies.

Let's take a closer look at studies that evaluate the effect of a particular drug or intervention. Consider, for example, that you want to evaluate the effect of a drug for hypertension. What do clinical trials tell us, and what do observational studies tell us?

From the results obtained in clinical trials, it is possible to extract information about the effect that the drug can have under the best possible conditions (i.e., its maximum potential), the effect that we can obtain when the conditions (external interactions) are controlled. In this context, it is to be expected that, in clinical studies, the drug has been evaluated in people who did not have other pathologies, and who were possibly relatively young compared to the average age of people with hypertension. The scientific validity of the data is excellent, as they come from a controlled study, but their external validity, i.e., their applicability in a broader context, may be difficult.

From the results obtained in real-world studies, or observational studies, it will be possible to extract information about the effect of the same drug when taken by people in their daily lives, i.e., under the real conditions in which this occurs, which means that the person may have several diseases at the same time and may or may not take the drug as recommended. The external validity of these studies is good or even excellent, but their internal validity may be reduced due to the many variables that can interfere with the observed effect.

Although I cannot state that experimental studies provide more scientific evidence than observational studies, what I would advise when evaluating a particular drug or health intervention is to analyze both types of studies and understand their limitations and strengths in terms of internal validity (methodology) and external validity (extrapolation of data to the population). The analysis of the results of both types of studies will allow you to know what the expected effect is under ideal conditions, but also how much this effect can be altered under conditions closer to reality.

Section III - How to Design a Clinical Study

Chapter 7 - Protocol Structure

When thinking about designing a new clinical research study, whether experimental or observational, the first thing you should think about is writing a protocol. The protocol is a document that should describe in detail the study's objectives, methodology, population, and procedures, allowing anyone to understand and reproduce it, as well as ensuring the recording of any methodological or other changes that occur after the study begins. In addition to ensuring the reproducibility of the study, the protocol seeks to ensure that, by defining the "rules" before the study begins, no (unplanned) procedures or analyses are carried out that are intended to modify or condition the results.

Protocols vary widely, depending on the characteristics of the study itself, but also on the research team. In the future, you should try to define the protocol structure that you identify with the most, but for now, I will present a basic structure that can serve as a model for you:

Title and Cover Page

Date and Version

Sponsor

Research Team

Research Centers

1. Synopsis
2. Acronyms and Abbreviations
3. Introduction and Rationale
4. Objectives

    4.1 Primary Objective

    4.2 Secondary Objectives

5. Endpoints

    5.1 Primary Endpoint

    5.2 Secondary Endpoints

6. Study Design
7. Participants

    7.1 Population

    7.2 Eligibility Criteria

    7.3 Early Withdrawal

    7.4 Study Termination

8. Procedures

    8.1 Recruitment

    8.2 Follow-up

    8.3 Treatments (may include details of the experimental medication, if it is a clinical trial)

    8.4 Randomization and Blinding (if applicable)

9. Safety/Adverse Events

    9.1 Definitions

    9.2 How to Assess and Record Adverse Events

10. Sampling

11. Statistical Analysis

    11.1 Analyzed Populations

    11.2 Variables

    11.3 Descriptive Analysis

    11.4 Primary Objective Analysis

    11.5 Secondary Objectives Analysis

    11.6 Safety Parameters Analysis

    11.7 Missing Data

    11.8 Protocol Deviations

12. Data Management

13. Monitoring

14. Ethical Considerations

    14.1 Confidentiality and Data Protection

    14.2 Declaration of Helsinki

    14.3 National Legislation and Good Clinical Practices

    14.4 Informed Consent

15. Publication Policy

16. Timeline

17. Table of Study Assessments

18. References

19. Appendices

The protocol usually has an initial page with the title, acronym if available, date, and version. This page should include the study registration number, if any, and the sponsoring organization, that is, who is responsible for the study. The organization responsible for the study can be, for example, a pharmaceutical sector company, a university, a research institute, a research team, or an individual.

The synopsis is, as the name suggests, a summary of the main aspects of the protocol. Although it does not have a predefined number of pages, as a reference, it can be considered between two and five pages, sometimes presented in table format (Figure 5).

On the Acronyms and Abbreviations page, you should include a comprehensive list of all acronyms and abbreviations used in the protocol text. By including this page, you will not need to define them throughout the text. For example, it may be useful to include a page with the units of measurement used in clinical analyses.

Figure 5: Example of the synopsis structure in table format.

Title	Title of the study and acronym or subtitle if applicable
Research Team	Names and affiliations
Date and Version	Date the protocol was approved. Version number if there are several before final approval
Centers (research sites)	Where participants will be recruited and other spaces where the study may take place, such as a central laboratory
Rationale	One or two paragraphs on the justification for conducting the study
Objectives	Description of the primary and secondary objectives (as described in the body of the protocol)
Study Design	Identification of the type of study, if it is a clinical trial indicate the phase of the study, the type of design (e.g., parallel or cross-over), whether it is randomized and the degree of concealment. For observational studies, indicate whether it is retrospective, cross-sectional or prospective and the study design.
Participants (eligibility criteria)	Indicate the length of the recruitment and follow-up period.
Procedures (summary)	Description of the inclusion and exclusion criteria
Sample	A summary of the procedures that will take place during the study, in the recruitment and follow-up phase, for example the scales to be

	applied, clinical information or the results of laboratory tests or imaging exams.
Statistical analysis	Brief rationale and sample size
Publications	A brief description of the type of analysis, particularly with a view to the main objective
Timeline	Indication of the publication plan

On the Acronyms and Abbreviations page, you should include a comprehensive list of all acronyms and abbreviations used in the protocol text. By including this page, you will not need to define them throughout the text. For example, it may be useful to include a page with the units of measurement used in clinical analyses.

The Introduction and Rationale chapter refers to the study's structure. Here you should present a summary of the current knowledge on the topic and the main studies (and bibliographic references) that have already been carried out on the subject. You should start with the more general aspects and then move on to the more specific conditions. The rationale refers to the reason for conducting the study and should be clear about the reasons behind it, that is, it should reflect the extent to which the results obtained will contribute to scientific progress and to a better clinical approach.

In the Objectives chapter, you should clearly and unambiguously describe the main objective of the study and its secondary objectives. Remember that, whenever possible, studies should have a single primary objective. The objectives can be presented in bullet point format, which facilitates reading. In terms of form, it is important to keep in mind that each objective should be independent and not depend on the understanding of previous objectives. Another aspect to consider is the way of writing, that is, if you use nouns or verbs, for example, if you use "characterization", "comparison" for one objective, you should not have another objective that starts with "comparing" or "describing".

The chapter on the definition of endpoints can come right after the objectives chapter or be presented later in the text, before the statistics chapter. In this chapter, you should detail for each objective how it will be measured. For example, if your objective is to assess quality of life, the endpoint should specify which scale will be used and how it will be evaluated/scored (a value on a continuous scale is used or the scale is transformed into categories). If the objective is described as "comparing the efficacy of...", the outcome should indicate what is meant by "efficacy".

In the Study Design chapter, the methodological characteristics should be presented. It should be indicated whether it is an intervention study and specified that it is a clinical trial. In the case of an observational study, you should indicate whether it is prospective, retrospective, or cross-sectional and, if prospective or retrospective (longitudinal studies), how long the follow-up period lasted. In terms of the study design itself, it may be "a cohort" (a single group of participants) or it may be a "cohort study", comparing several groups of participants, which can be separated into groups based on the presence of a risk factor, a demographic or clinical characteristic or, for example, exposure to a certain drug. Note that observational studies can NEVER be randomized or blinded; these are techniques that can only be used in interventional studies.

In the case of an interventional study, you should describe whether it is a clinical trial (a situation in which the intervention is the use of an experimental drug, evaluating its efficacy, safety and/or pharmacokinetics and/or pharmacodynamics). If it is a clinical trial, the study phase should be indicated. Interventional studies are prospective by definition, so there is no need to mention this fact in the protocol text. The intervention and control should be indicated. It should also mention whether any randomization technique will be used to distribute participants among study groups and whether it is planned to be blinded.

Regarding the specifics of the study design, you should mention the duration of follow-up of the participants and the type of design, that is, the study structure, for example, whether it is a parallel study, a crossover study, an adaptive design, etc. (see details in a later chapter).

In the chapter entitled Participants, you should include a first part in which you explain the general characteristics of the people who will be able to participate in the study. Then list the inclusion and exclusion criteria. These criteria should be comprehensive and clear so that they are easy to understand and apply. The inclusion and exclusion criteria should not be presented negatively (that is, if you say, as an inclusion criterion, that participants must be 18 years of age or older, you should not say, as an exclusion criterion, that participants should not be under 18 years of age). Although inclusion and exclusion criteria are specific to each study, in most of them it is part of these criteria to mention the existence of written informed consent.

Still in the chapter on participants, you should refer, if applicable, to the reasons that may lead to premature withdrawal from the study and how these situations will be handled (which information will be used and how, and whether specific procedures will be carried out). You should also refer to the criteria for study termination.

The chapter entitled Procedures explains the duration of the recruitment period (during which new people can participate in the study) and the assessments that are part of the participant selection and inclusion process. It also explains how follow-up is conducted, its duration, and the procedures that are performed, for example, laboratory analyses, imaging tests, application of scales, or evaluation of side effects. In the case of an intervention study, particularly a clinical trial, it should include a subchapter describing the experimental drug, including the data available on the experimental product from previous studies (pharmacokinetics, pharmacodynamics, efficacy, and safety), the dose and frequency of use, the route of administration, and any precautions.

In the case of a randomized study, the randomization method and the groups evaluated should be described. In the case of a blinded study, it should be described whether the study is single, double, or triple blind and exactly who has access to what, especially in the case of a serious adverse effect that requires the opening of blind codes and knowledge of the drug administered.

In the chapter on safety/adverse events, you should present the definitions of "adverse event", "serious adverse event", and the definitions of causality as defined in the Glossary of Good Clinical Practice Standards (15). This chapter should describe how adverse events occurring during the study will be collected and reported.

In the Sampling chapter, you should describe whether or not the study is testing a formal hypothesis. If so, the sample size should be calculated such that the hypothesis can be proven, if confirmed, or rejected, if not. You should present the clinical and statistical assumptions considered, including the study power and significance level. The clinical assumptions, for example, for the expected success rate in a given therapeutic group, should be justified based on other published studies, which should be referenced in the protocol text.

If dropouts are anticipated during the study (participants who do not complete the study), this should be accounted for in the sample size calculation, and the expected dropout rate and re-calculation of the sample size should be mentioned taking this into account.

In the case of a descriptive study, you should base the sample size calculation on the assumed margin of error for the intervals to be presented, or define it as a convenience sample, taking into account the target population.

In the Statistical Analysis chapter, you should include a description of the populations to be analyzed, in case multiple populations are considered. For example, in a given study, you may consider that the data will be analyzed for all people who started the study, for all people who reached the end of the study per protocol, and for all people who took the test drug at least once. In this case, three populations would be analyzed.

You should start by presenting the variables to be analyzed in the study, indicating what type of variable it is (continuous, ordinal, categorical) and whether it is a variable collected at baseline or throughout the study and, if so, when.

The protocol should describe the techniques that will be used to descriptively analyze the variables. Next, it should describe the techniques used to make comparisons between groups and comparisons between variables, whether bivariate or multivariate. The techniques should be described to meet each of the objectives presented at the beginning. The significance level considered for the analyses to be performed should be mentioned.

You should individually describe how you will analyze the safety parameters.

In the statistical analysis chapter, you should also describe how missing data and protocol deviation situations will be handled (for example, the value of a laboratory analysis that was performed outside the protocol execution timeframe, e.g., it should have been performed 20-30 days after the previous assessment and was performed 35 days after the assessment). If one or more interim analyses (data analyses performed during the study) are planned, they should be justified and should describe what will be analyzed.

In the Data Management chapter, you should describe how the database will be created and stored, who has access to what information, and what is the level of security for those accesses. You should also describe if there are procedures to ensure the validity and consistency of the recorded data, who is responsible for executing them, and at what point.

In the chapter titled Monitoring, describe how the study is monitored (if applicable), i.e., if there are professionals on the team that validate the coherence and consistency of the data recorded in the data collection notebooks (electronic or paper). If the data is monitored, you should describe what data is monitored and how frequently.

In the Ethical (or Ethical and Regulatory) Considerations chapter, you should describe how confidentiality, privacy, and anonymity of data are ensured.

You should mention that the study was conducted in accordance with the Declaration of Helsinki (18) and that it is in compliance with national legislation and Good Clinical Practice Standards. This chapter should also include a reference to the existence of the written informed consent and the participant information sheet, which should be appended. In the case of a study where a waiver of informed consent will be requested, this should be mentioned and its applicability justified.

The Publication Policy chapter should describe how the study results will be communicated, including presentations at conferences, scientific publications, and other forms of dissemination.

The protocol should include a Timeline chapter, listing the key dates, such as: study start, date of first participant inclusion, date of last assessment of last participant, recruitment period, follow-up period, database lock, data analysis (interim and final), and publication.

It is useful to include a table of assessments throughout the study. This table should list in the first column all the assessments that will be carried out, including: informed consent signature, demographic data collection, clinical evaluation, laboratory tests, imaging tests, scales, among others. The headers of the other columns should show the different study assessment time points, for example: baseline assessment, 3-month, 6-month and 12-month/study end assessment. The body of the table should be filled by marking with an "X" the assessments that occur at each of the assessment time points (also commonly referred to as study visit).

The last chapters are the Bibliographic References and the Appendices. The latter may include any documents that the research team deems relevant, including, for example, the participant information sheet, the informed consent statement, and/or the scales or questionnaires to be used.

As I mentioned at the beginning of this chapter, there is no single model for a protocol, as it depends on the type of study and should be done specifically by the study team. In addition to the model presented above, I suggest that you take a look at some of the clinical study protocols presented on the platform https://clinicaltrials.gov/ (19) to see other alternatives and examples.

On this platform, you can enter a disease or condition of interest to search for studies, select the "Study Documents" option on the right sidebar, and then select "Study Protocols", which will display only those studies for which a version of the protocol is available for reading.

Chapter 8 - Research Question

Every research project starts with a question. Questioning is the cornerstone of discovery and the pursuit of new answers. In this context, you will not be surprised if I tell you that clinical studies should also start with one or more research questions. Studies usually begin with a general research question, which is subdivided into more specific questions.

The research question, or initial question, reflects the main question that the study will attempt to answer. In most situations, the research question gives rise to the primary objective of the study, although it can also directly give rise to several of the secondary objectives, depending on the degree of complexity and scope of the question itself.

The research question should be written in the study protocol and, since it is a question, it should be written in an interrogative form. Technically, the research question should have some specific characteristics: it should be clear, unambiguous, relevant, feasible, and ethical. (20).

We consider a question to be clear if you can easily understand what you want to study. On the other hand, it is unambiguous if, in addition to being perceptible, it is understood in the same way by anyone who reads it. There are questions that, although clear, can be interpreted differently by those who read them, for example, because they contain words with a certain degree of ambiguity.

A relevant question is one that effectively attempts to answer a problem or a doubt. Sometimes, there are research questions that are not really questions, that is, before starting the study, you already know what the answer to the question will be, because similar studies have already been carried out and the proposed study does not add anything new to your knowledge. You should avoid this type of situation. However, you should assume that it may be relevant to carry out a study similar to one that has already been done, if it evaluates a different population, or is carried out in a different geographical region, or simply if you want to update the data. Rarely is a study completely new; in most situations, studies try to add some information to what we already know.

When evaluating a research question for a clinical study, it is necessary to consider its feasibility and ethics. The question presented should be answerable, that is, you should design a study that can be methodologically sound, but for which you foresee major (insurmountable) difficulties in carrying out. At the same time, it should always be considered whether the proposed study is ethical, that is, one should never forget that the individual rights of the participants always take precedence over the research itself.

There are several ways to frame a research question. One of the most commonly used, for studies designed to evaluate the effects of a drug or intervention, is the following structure (21), later transformed into PICOT (22).

        P - Population or Problem

        I – Intervention

        C – Comparison

        O - Outcome

The PICO structure has undergone some changes and interpretations, so that "P" can also denote "Problem" and "I" can denote "Condition of interest" or "Indicator under study".

A new structure called PICOT has also been proposed, in which the introduction of the letter "T" includes the concept of "Time". The PICOT structure has also been proposed in the form of PICOT-D, which includes "Data" (23).

In addition to these methodological structures, there are numerous others, such as "Exposure", "Pre-existing conditions", "Type of study", "Study design", "Duration" or "Context" (24).

More important than choosing one structure or another is to consider which elements are most relevant to clearly explain what you want to study. From a global point of view, you can accept that the research question defines what will be studied, who will be studied, and how it will be studied.

In simple terms, you can subdivide the questions (for quantitative studies) into (25):

- Descriptive, related to a disease or risk factor.

- Evaluation of an intervention/treatment (comparison).

- Etiologic or causal.

- Descriptive, related to a diagnostic means.

- Evaluation of a diagnostic means (comparison).

- Scale validation.

- Prognostic evaluation.

- Evaluation of survival time.

If you want to describe a disease, you can ask the following question, for example:

"What is the annual prevalence of breast cancer in women aged 80 and over in the United States in the last 5 years?"

The most important aspects to consider when structuring your research question are:

Population - women aged 80 and over.

Disease of interest - breast cancer.

Outcome/measure - annual prevalence.

Time: last 5 years.

Location: United States.

But if you want to compare the effect of two drugs, the question should have different characteristics, for example:

"In transgender individuals receiving gender-affirming hormone therapy, is drug A more effective in reducing the area of skin lesions than drug B in the treatment of psoriasis after 6 months of treatment?"

Population: transgender individuals receiving gender-affirming hormone therapy.

Intervention: drug A for the treatment of psoriasis.

Comparison: drug B for the treatment of psoriasis.

Outcome/measure - efficacy: reduction in skin lesion area.

Time - 6 months of treatment.

Consider another example, regarding a question created to evaluate prognostic factors:

"Are sexual orientation, gender identity, socioeconomic status, family history, and smoking status associated with the risk of death from prostate cancer in cisgender men seen in a hospital urology or oncology clinic in the last 5 years?"

> Population - cisgender men seen in a hospital urology or oncology clinic.
>
> Exposure/prognostic factor - sexual orientation, gender identity, socioeconomic status, family history, smoking status.
>
> Outcome/measure - (risk of) death.
>
> Time: 5 years.

As an example, consider some poorly structured research questions:

"What is the impact of belonging to a sexual and/or gender minority on mental health?

The question is poorly structured - why? It analyzes the different components in isolation:

> Study population - people belonging to a sexual and/or gender minority; although not very specific, the definition allows us to understand which people will be included in the study - correct.
>
> As this is not a treatment or intervention study, it would not make sense to apply the PICO methodology, assuming "intervention" and "comparator", therefore, you should consider "condition of interest".
>
> Condition of interest - described as mental health; although the context is understood, it is too vague and too broad - incorrect (it could be explained, for example, as level of anxiety or prevalence of depression).

Outcome - described as "impact". This is the type of word that should not be used in this context. It is ambiguous and unclear. Although in colloquial language the meaning can be understood, in scientific and methodological terms it does not explain what is being measured and what outcome is being analyzed: incorrect.

Time - the question does not refer to the time period of the analysis (or date), which is relevant in the context.

"In the last 10 years, has there been an increase in the incidence of major cardiovascular events in transgender individuals?"

This research question is poorly structured. It analyzes the different components in isolation:

Study population: transgender individuals, allows us to understand which people will be included in the study. Considering the clinical context of the question, it might make sense to specify whether they are individuals who are undergoing hormone treatment or not, but this specificity can be defined in the protocol.

Condition of interest - major cardiovascular events; clear and well defined, it could be specified in more detail in the objectives what is meant by "major".

Outcome - described as "increased frequency of major cardiovascular events". This is an outcome with a binary answer: yes or no. This type of yes/no question should not be used as a research question in a clinical study because it is too reductionist. The question can be addressed and answered, but it should be framed in a broader scope that allows the information collected to be useful for clinical practice.

Time - last 10 years.

Chapter 9 - Objectives and Endpoints

In a clinical study, you should define the objectives according to your research question. Depending on the aspect you consider most relevant, you should specify a primary objective and, if possible, only one. In other words, the primary objective answers the research question and defines the most appropriate study design to answer it. Additionally, based on the primary objective, you can define the hypotheses to calculate the necessary sample size for the study.

Secondary objectives are usually more than one and aim to explore aspects of the research that the primary objective does not answer, or to analyze subgroups of the study population. In some situations, secondary objectives allow the evaluation of new hypotheses that may lead to new clinical studies.

The types of objectives in a clinical study are similar to those described for research questions. Thus, we have the following objectives:

- Descriptive

- Analytical - Comparison between groups of people

- Analytical - Association between variables

- Analytical - Prognostic analysis

- Analytical - Survival analysis

Studies whose main objective is descriptive may focus on determining the frequency of an event, such as prevalence, incidence, lethality studies, among others, or on characterizing a specific population, which may correspond to a population with a particular disease, a population exposed to an event, a population with a risk factor, or a population to which a specific drug or therapeutic intervention is administered. Examples include:

- Determining the prevalence of smoking among people belonging to sexual minorities in 2022 in the United States.

- Characterizing cardiovascular risk in women over 65 years of age in 2023 in the United States.

- Characterizing sleep patterns in people medicated with serotonin reuptake inhibitor antidepressants for more than 12 months.

Studies whose main objective is to compare outcomes between two (or more) groups of people may, for example, analyze the response to two drugs (the tested drug versus the comparator, the comparator can be another drug or, if it is a clinical trial, it can also be a placebo). This type of study may also aim to compare a group of people exposed and not exposed to a particular event, or to evaluate the occurrence of a disease in two groups of people with different characteristics, for example, different gender identities, sex, or age. Examples include:

- Comparing the prevalence of eating disorders between cisgender and transgender youth aged 12 to 16 years in the United States over the past five years.

- Comparing the time to peak absorption of an oral antidiabetic drug in people aged 55 to 65 years and in people over 65 years of age.

- Comparing the efficacy (reduction in the number of attacks) of treatment A versus treatment B for the prevention of migraines in transgender men receiving gender-affirming hormone therapy.

Studies aimed at analyzing the association between two or more variables seek to determine whether the variables in question influence each other, positively or negatively, or whether the behavior of one variable is not related to one or more variables. Examples include:

- Evaluating the relationship between age and hemoglobin value in people over 50 years of age.

- Associating educational level with stress scale scores in sexual and/or gender minorities.

Studies that analyze prognosis (or risk) attempt to explain a particular variable (called the dependent variable), for example, "good prognosis," through a set of other variables (independent variables). Examples include:

- Evaluating variables that predict success in lesbian women undergoing in vitro fertilization (IVF).

- Evaluating variables associated with the occurrence of suicide attempts in women with postpartum depression.

Studies that aim to analyze survival analyze the occurrence of the situation in question over time, estimating a probability curve. This can be survival in the strict sense of the word or, more broadly, include studies that analyze, for example, disease progression, time to event occurrence, or time to treatment persistence. Examples include:

- Evaluating median survival in women with stage IV breast cancer over 70 years of age.

- Evaluating treatment persistence time for smoking cessation in transgender men undergoing gender-affirming hormone therapy.

The term endpoint refers to how the objective is measured. Whenever you define a primary or secondary outcome, you should define the associated endpoint.

There are situations in which the endpoint is directly derived from the objective, making them seem like the same thing. For example, if the objective is "To determine the prevalence of smoking among people belonging to sexual minorities in the United States in 2022," the endpoint will be "prevalence of smoking among people belonging to sexual minorities in the United States in 2022."

In other circumstances, the objective does not directly infer what the parameter is. For example, consider a study whose objective is "Comparison of the efficacy of treatment A versus treatment B for the prevention of migraine in transgender men receiving gender-affirming hormone therapy." In this case, we need to define how efficacy will be evaluated, that is, the best way to quantify this objective. For example, you could say that efficacy is evaluated by the "percentage reduction in the number of migraines over a given period of time." But you could also have chosen as an endpoint for the same study "the percentage of people who had fewer than six attacks during a 12-month treatment period," or any other clinically relevant assessment.

If you determine that a particular objective is evaluated by more than one endpoint, you should make this clear in the protocol. You can choose to maintain a single objective or split it into multiple objectives, depending on the different outcomes associated with it.

In certain situations, it may be useful to define a composite endpoint. A composite endpoint is one that combines several different conditions. For example, in the study mentioned above, it could have been stipulated that it would be considered effective if people had a simultaneous reduction of more than 75% in the number of migraines before the study and fewer than 1 migraine per month for 12 months.

In some situations, it is useful to use surrogate endpoints. Surrogate endpoints are those that evaluate the objective through markers (variables) that give an indirect idea of what we are measuring (25, 26). Surrogate endpoints are, for example, tumor markers or biomarkers, which allow making inferences about disease activity (27).

You should choose to use surrogate endpoints whenever it is not possible to directly evaluate what you want to assess, either because of technical difficulties, cost, or time. Surrogate endpoints need validation, that is, a demonstration that their variation (their value) is directly related to what you want to evaluate (28,29). For example, forced expiratory volume in the first second (FEV1) is considered a surrogate parameter for evaluating acute bronchospasm and is accepted for evaluating the efficacy of beta-2 adrenergic receptor agonists. In cancer, progression-free survival (PFS) is accepted as a surrogate marker for evaluating the administered therapy, assuming that it has a direct relationship with tumor activity and, consequently, with survival. Another example is the use of glycated hemoglobin (HbA1c) as a biomarker to evaluate glycemic control in people with type 2 diabetes.

Chapter 10 - Study Designs

The following sections - interventional clinical trials and observational studies - describe in detail the different types of studies and the methodological characteristics inherent to each design. In this introductory chapter, I would like to present a brief overview of the different types of study designs and their suitability in relation to the defined objectives.

In general terms, and as we have already seen, clinical studies can be classified into studies with intervention, known as interventional studies or experimental studies, in which the standard clinical practice is modified, and studies without intervention, known as observational studies.

An interventional clinical study is any research that advocates a change, influence, or programming of health care, behavior, or knowledge of participants or caregivers, with the objective of discovering or verifying effects on health, including exposure to drugs, use of medical devices, performing surgical techniques, exposure to radiotherapy, application of cosmetic and body hygiene products, physiotherapeutic intervention, psychotherapeutic intervention, use of transfusions, cell therapy, participation in individual or group educational sessions, diet intervention, intervention in health care access or organization, or intervention designated as unconventional therapy.

A non-interventional or observational clinical study is a study in which the following conditions are met:

- Drugs are prescribed or medical devices are used according to the conditions established in the marketing authorization or in the conformity assessment procedure, respectively;

- The inclusion of participants in a specific therapeutic strategy is not predetermined by a study protocol but depends on current practice;

- The decision to prescribe the drug or use a medical device is clearly dissociated from the decision to include or not the person in the study;

- No other complementary diagnostic or evaluation procedure is applied to participants and epidemiological methods are used to analyze the collected data.

When defining the design of a clinical study, you should start by stating whether it is a study with or without intervention (specifying if it is a clinical trial, if applicable).

Continuing with the topic of study design, you should indicate the time period of the study, i.e., whether it is a cross-sectional or longitudinal study. Cross-sectional studies are those in which each participant is assessed at a single point in time, with no intention of assessing over time.

Longitudinal studies follow people over time, whether short or long, and can be retrospective or prospective. In retrospective studies, information is collected over time, but the study time point is in the past compared to when the protocol was developed and data collected. In prospective studies, information is also collected over time, but the data collection occurs in the future compared to when the protocol was developed.

For example, you may be designing a retrospective study in which you want to assess overall survival until the end of last year in women smokers with advanced lung cancer diagnosed in 2017. The protocol and data collection are being conducted now, but the data refers to the period from 2017 until the participant's death or, at most, until the end of last year.

I could have designed the same type of study prospectively. In that case, I could have assessed overall survival in women smokers with advanced lung cancer, diagnosed from the start of the study and followed for up to 5 years. The protocol would be conducted now, data collection would begin in 6 months, for example, and follow-up would be until the participant's death or up to 5 years after the end of the recruitment period.

What are the main differences between the two designs?

If you opted for a retrospective study, you have the great advantage that the data collection period is short and, consequently, the results are fast. The data already exists (in the clinical records), so the study time is limited by the time needed to approve the study, the time spent on retrospective analysis of the records and on data collection. The disadvantages of this design are mainly related to the availability and quality of the data. Another aspect to take into account is whether or not there have been therapeutic or other advances that have led to the prediction that the survival of these patients will be very different in the last five years than what is currently expected.

If a prospective study is chosen, it has the enormous advantage that the data collection is planned and, therefore, more complete and reliable. On the other hand, there is the time limitation, i.e., the study will take at least 6 months to be able to start recruiting and another 5 years, which was the maximum period established for follow-up. In addition, there is the period for study presentation and approval at the participating centers and the data analysis period.

As an example, it can be considered that the retrospective study described above would last (from protocol to final report) 18 months, while the prospective study would last (from protocol to final report) 7 years.

Finally, I would like to point out that intervention studies are always prospective, for obvious reasons arising from the implementation of the intervention.

In summary, you should keep in mind that, in terms of design, a study can be with or without intervention and, in the latter case, it can be cross-sectional or longitudinal, prospective or retrospective. In addition to these aspects, you should mention in the study design whether it is a descriptive or comparative study and, in that case, between how many groups. You should also mention if it is a situation where the groups being compared are matched groups, either because it is a case-control study or because it is a matched cohort study (see details in the respective chapters).

Another point to be mentioned is whether the study is community-based, hospital-based, primary care unit-based or other type of study, whether it is national or international in scope, and whether it is single-center or multicenter.

Chapter 11 - Population

Correctly defining the characteristics of the population that may participate in a given study is critical to its success. Therefore, this is one of the most important things to think about when you are part of a clinical study design team.

Obviously, the population to be included in a given study depends on the study objectives. However, under the pretext of making the sample to be studied more homogeneous and, thus, increasing the internal validity of our study (better controlling for external variables that may influence the results), we systematically leave out many population groups, including LGBTQIA+ people, people of different origins, ancestry or skin color, but also the elderly and people with various diseases or who are polymedicated.

When defining which individuals are eligible for a study, think about which characteristics are vital to be able to assess the objectives to be achieved and consider excluding only situations that may pose a risk to the participants themselves or that directly interfere with what is intended to be evaluated.

Age and sex (sex assigned at birth) are two of the most cross-cutting characteristics in the constitution of inclusion and exclusion criteria for clinical studies. Let's take a look at each of them:

Age - It is common to define whether the study can include children or only adults. Some studies are more specific and define a lower and upper age limit.

The definition of an upper limit for the age of people who can be included may be due to specific study contingencies, but, in most cases, it is due to the bias that older people should not participate in clinical studies or simply to the technical difficulty of dealing with confounding variables, such as polymedication or the presence of several concomitant pathologies. What is certain is that, in the case of clinical studies, most of the drugs being evaluated will actually be consumed by the elderly, who have the greatest burden of disease. So the question arises as to whether it makes sense to leave out of the study population the individuals who will later be the target of the intervention being evaluated. By not including the elderly in clinical studies, it is assumed that the dose, absorption, metabolization or elimination of a drug can be extrapolated to any individual, even though the studies were conducted in young and, probably, male individuals.

When defining the age criteria for individuals who can participate in a study, it is important to consider whether, in the absence of a strict impediment or contraindication, it is more ethical to include the elderly and very elderly.

As for the inclusion of children and youth, they are usually only included in studies on situations that directly affect them. In other words, pathologies and drugs that affect both adults and youth are, most of the time, evaluated only in the adult population. The non-inclusion of young people under 18 years of age is usually justified by the simplification of processes, as their inclusion requires specific ethical requirements, especially in terms of informed consent. As I mentioned with the elderly, in the case of young people it is important to assess whether they are being protected when they are not included in a study or whether they are being discriminated against.

Sex (sex assigned at birth): Most studies on diseases that are not specific to women or men tend to include people of both sexes. In the eligibility criteria, you can explicitly mention "people" or "individuals".

Despite the trend towards greater equity in recent years, there is still an asymmetry in the inclusion of women in Phase 1 clinical studies (see Chapter 17).

An important point to note is that when "sex" is mentioned in the eligibility criteria of a study, it refers to sex assigned at birth and not gender identity. In other words, when a study mentions that it includes individuals of both sexes and says nothing about gender identity, it must be recognized that it may include both cisgender female and male individuals as well as non-binary gender individuals. If it is necessary to exclude a certain group, this must be explicit and duly justified.

For example, if you are conducting a study in which you do not want to include people who are on hormone therapy, this should be explicitly written in the selection criteria, and not that transgender people are excluded, as one thing does not necessarily imply the other.

Chapter 12 - Methodology and Procedures

When we talk about the methodology of a clinical study, we are encompassing all the points mentioned above, that is, the definition of the study design and the study population are part of the methodology and, in a broader sense, even the definition of the outcomes can be considered part of the methodology. In this chapter, we will look at how the study is conducted, that is, the journey of each participant, with all the activities that this implies.

In the study protocol, it is necessary to clearly define which procedures will be applied and what type of instruments/measures will be used. There are studies for which it is very easy to define the procedures. For example, imagine that you are going to conduct a cross-sectional observational study in which you will apply a questionnaire to the general population about the level of knowledge and acceptance of vaccines. What are the procedures for this study?

- It is a single assessment.

- It is a self-completed questionnaire (on paper), to be administered at home (in a door-to-door questionnaire approach).

- It takes about 5 minutes to complete.

- The questionnaire consists of 35 questions, all of them closed-ended.

- The selection of households is done in advance using procedures defined to calculate the representativeness of the sample, detailed in the corresponding chapter of the study protocol (which we will address later).

- After the data is collected, it is entered into a database.

The points above describe how the study will be conducted and the instrument (in this case, a questionnaire) to be used. The procedures are: the application of a self-completed paper questionnaire, which is carried out door-to-door, at the residence, and the instrument applied is a closed-response questionnaire, applied on paper, with a completion time of about 5 minutes.

Although the procedures and instruments in the example above are simple, when we think of a prospective longitudinal study or, even more so, a clinical trial, the procedures can be extraordinarily complex. Let's now imagine that a study is conducted on a new antidiabetic drug, in which it is compared to a control drug. Let's say it is a 6-month randomized clinical trial evaluating efficacy, safety, and quality of life. What procedures and instruments should you describe?

- At the first visit (a visit is the moment of contact between the participant and the research team, for example, a medical consultation), which we will call the screening visit, the research team identifies adults with type 2 diabetes (defined according to the study's eligibility criteria), explains the study to them and invites them to participate. After they agree and sign an informed consent form, data is collected for demographic and clinical characterization, and laboratory tests are requested to verify compliance with the inclusion criteria and to serve as baseline values.

Here it must be described what information will be collected for demographic and clinical characterization and which laboratory tests will be performed.

- Between 7 and 15 days after the screening visit, the initial visit (visit 1) will take place. After confirmation of the eligibility criteria, the participant is randomly assigned by an automated system to one of the two study groups and to one of the drugs (experimental or control drug). The values of the tests performed are recorded. A clinical examination, an electrocardiogram (ECG) and the EQ-5D quality of life scale (30) are applied. Each person is given a diary and it is explained to them that they should record any symptoms (adverse effects) that arise in the period between this assessment and the next one within 4 weeks (with a date flexibility of plus or minus 3 days). New laboratory tests are requested 3 days before the next visit.

Here you must describe what information will be collected in the clinical examination, how the electrocardiogram (ECG) will be performed and what laboratory tests will be requested. The EQ-5D scale and the content of the diary that the person will take home should be described.

In clinical trials, the dates of the assessments are usually very strict and an interval of days is stipulated within which the visit must be performed. This interval is called a "window" and depends on the time between visits. If this interval is short, the flexibility window will be smaller, while if the interval between visits is long, the window will also be larger.

• At visit 2 (4 weeks ± 3 days), a clinical examination is performed, tests and any adverse events, reported by the individual or recorded in the diary, are evaluated and recorded. Medication and a new diary are given. New laboratory tests are requested 3 days before the next visit. A new visit is scheduled for 8 weeks later (with a date flexibility of plus or minus 5 days).

• At visit 3 (12 weeks ± 5 days), a clinical examination is performed, the tests performed are evaluated and recorded, as well as any adverse events, whether reported by the individual or recorded in the diary. The EQ-5D quality of life scale is applied. The medications and a new diary are provided. New laboratory tests are requested 3 days before the next visit. A new visit (final visit) is scheduled for 12 weeks later (with a date flexibility of approximately 5 days).

• At visit 4, the final visit (at 24 weeks ± 5 days), a clinical examination, an ECG and the tests performed, as well as any adverse events reported by the individual or recorded in the diary, are evaluated and recorded. The EQ-5D quality of life scale is applied.

You must anticipate that the person may withdraw from the study at any time (without having to give any justification). In this case, you should ask the person to complete the details of the so-called early discontinuation/withdrawal visit, if they accept. The person may or may not agree and may or may not be available to do everything planned for that visit, which is usually similar to the final visit.

In studies like this one (and in much more complex studies), it is useful to prepare a summary table of the assessments at each visit, as shown in Figure 6.

In addition to the items above, part of the description of the procedures involves explaining how the research team will select potential participants at each site, for example, in a specific consultation, in the emergency room or in a specific ward.

It should be clearly stated how long it will take to recruit the participating people, indicating the start and end date of recruitment and the duration of the follow-up period. For example, in the study described above, you can consider a 12-month recruitment period (time to include all the people needed to obtain the sample calculated for this study) and 24 weeks of follow-up (the follow-up time is for each person included and is counted from the date of inclusion).

Another important sub-chapter in the methodology is the detailed description of the tests requested, for example, requested analyses, imaging methods or other complementary tests should be described. If the test in question is not standardized, the complete method to be applied must be written.

Figure 6 - Summary table of assessments performed during the study.

	Screening visit	V1 Initiation visit	V2 4 weeks ± 3 days	V3 12 weeks ± 5 days	V4 24 weeks ± 5 days	Withdrawal visit
Eligibility assessment	X	X				
Randomization		X				
Informed consent	X					
Demographic data	X					
Clinical data	X					
Clinical examination		X	X	X	X	X
ECG		X	X	X	X	X
Laboratory tests		X				
EQ-5D scale		X		X	X	X
Delivery of adverse event log		X	X	X		
Adverse event registration			X	X	X	X
Delivery of medication		X	X	X		

In the case of laboratory tests, you must explain whether they will be performed in the laboratories of the hospitals where the study is conducted, whether they will be performed outside, but in different locations, depending on the center, or whether there is a so-called "central laboratory". In this case, each center sends its samples to the same laboratory, which performs all the analyses. If this is the case, it must be informed how blood samples or other biological material are collected, whether they are subjected to any procedure, such as centrifugation, how they are packaged and sent to the central laboratory, including the entity responsible for transportation.

As mentioned above, all scales to be used must be described. It should be indicated that they have been validated for the population in question and the relevant bibliographic reference should be provided. The questions and types of responses should be described and how the scale is scored and classified.

In the case of studies with medicinal products and, in particular, clinical trials, the medicinal products themselves (experimental and control) must be described, as well as the way in which the randomization and, if applicable, blinding procedures are performed (explained in the chapters on Clinical Trials).

Chapter 13 - Ethical and Regulatory Framework

When thinking about conducting any clinical study, you must be aware of some documents that define the essential ethical and legal principles for your research, such as the Declaration of Helsinki (18), the Good Clinical Practice Guidelines (31) and the Clinical Research law of each country.

The Declaration of Helsinki was drafted in 1964 by the World Medical Association (WMA) as a statement of ethical principles for clinical research involving human subjects and has since been updated. Its text includes central aspects, such as the fundamental respect for human rights, and specific aspects related to clinical research, such as its risks and benefits, the technical and scientific quality of protocols, the inclusion of people belonging to vulnerable groups, ethics committees, informed consent, privacy and confidentiality of data and disclosure of results.

The Good Clinical Practice (GCP) guidelines are part of a set of guidelines provided by the International Council for Harmonisation (ICH). The ICH was created in 1990 by the International Federation of Pharmaceutical Manufacturers Associations (IFPMA) with the goal of harmonizing practices related to the evaluation of drugs and other medical products between Europe, Japan, and the United States. The GCP guidelines are part of an efficacy guideline, called ICH E6, and can be consulted in full at https://www.ich.org/page/efficacy-guidelines.

The scope of acceptance and application now extends beyond the initial countries to, for example, Brazil, Mexico, China, Canada, Egypt, Republic of Korea, Turkey, and Saudi Arabia.

The GCP document is divided into general principles, ethics committees, investigator team, sponsor organization, clinical study protocol, investigator's brochure, and essential documents for the conduct of a clinical study, outlining the responsibilities of each organization or person involved in the research and detailing how the documents must be executed.

One of the main aspects mentioned in the above documents is the fundamental respect for the rights of the human person, which takes precedence over the interests of science and society. In other words, before considering what is important for the clinical study, it is necessary to consider if this is in the best interest of the individual. A specific situation is that of the person who wishes to withdraw from the study. This may not be good for the study results, but if that is the person's will, it must be respected and even supported.

1 - Clinical studies are conducted with strict respect for the principle of human dignity and fundamental rights.

2 - The rights of clinical study participants always take precedence over the interests of science and society.

3 - In the conduct of clinical studies, all precautions must be taken to respect the privacy of the individual and minimize any damage to their personality rights and their physical and mental integrity.

Chapter 14 - Information for the participant and informed consent

All persons participating in clinical studies should be informed about the study's objectives, procedures, risks, and benefits. This information should be provided by the research team, assessing at all times whether the information is being understood by the person invited to participate and answering any questions that may arise. In addition to the oral explanation, the person invited to participate should receive the same information in writing, so that they can read it calmly and carefully before agreeing to participate in the study.

Only after the study has been explained in detail and the participating person has read the information sheet should the informed consent document be signed.

Informed consent can be defined as follows:

The express decision to participate in a clinical study, taken freely by a person with the capacity to do so or, in the absence of this, by their legal representative, after having been duly informed about the nature, scope, consequences and risks of the study, as well as about the right to withdraw from the study at any time, without consequences, according to the guidelines issued by the competent Ethics Committee, which must include the definition of the appropriate means of providing it, which must be in writing, if applicable.

A person who is participating in a clinical study may withdraw their informed consent at any time, without incurring any responsibility and without having to justify it. Furthermore, the withdrawal of consent does not require any special form and can be expressed or implied. Although informed consent is mandatory for all clinical studies, there are situations where it may not be required. The Ethics Committee responsible for evaluating the study may waive informed consent. For example, this could occur in a study considered relevant, which retrospectively evaluates data from people who have already died or who cannot be contacted at the time of the study. The withdrawal of consent must be requested from the Ethics Committee and duly justified.

For underage participants, consent must be given by a legal representative, and informed consent is also required from minors aged 16 or over. Minors should receive information about the study, their participation, risks and benefits in a manner appropriate to their age and ability to understand. Again, consent can be revoked at any time.

It is important to note that it is the responsibility of the research team to accommodate and respect the wishes of underage participants who are able to form an opinion and evaluate the information provided, particularly respecting their refusal to participate or leave the study.

For adult participants unable to give informed consent, note that the law implies that their participation in the study is only possible if the person who is now incapable of giving informed consent has not previously refused to participate in the study. If this is not the case, consent must be obtained from the person holding legal representation, and the person holding legal representation must presume the willingness of the person invited to participate in the study. It is the responsibility of the research team to ensure that this will is respected, taking into account the ability of the incapacitated person to assess the situation and give their opinion. As in the case of underage participants, information about the study, risks and benefits should also be provided in a manner appropriate to their ability to understand.

Section IV - Intervention Studies

Chapter 15 - Clinical Trial - Concept

A clinical trial can be defined as:

> Any research conducted on human subjects, designed to discover or verify the clinical, pharmacological or other pharmacodynamic effects of an investigational medicinal product, or to identify adverse effects of an investigational medicinal product, or to analyze the absorption, distribution, metabolism and elimination of an investigational medicinal product, with the objective of determining its safety or efficacy.

From this definition, it is important to keep in mind some critical aspects to consider a study as a clinical trial. First, it is important to note that the definition applies only to studies in humans and studies evaluating investigational medicinal products, which are understood as:

> The pharmaceutical form of an active substance or placebo, tested or used as a reference in a clinical trial, including medicinal products whose introduction to the market has been authorized, but which are used or prepared, in terms of pharmaceutical form or packaging, in a manner different from the authorized form, or used for an unauthorized indication or to obtain more information about the authorized form.

From this definition, an investigational medicinal product is one that is still under development, not yet marketed, but also one that, although marketed, is being used in a study outside the approved indication, at a different dose, formulation, population or route of administration. In other words, a medicinal product that is being used outside its marketing authorization (MA).

The definition of a clinical trial emphasizes that the purpose of the study should be to evaluate clinical, pharmacological or other pharmacodynamic effects, which translates into studies that assess efficacy, safety profile or tolerability (adverse events), pharmacokinetics or pharmacodynamics.

To conclude, I would like to emphasize that, by definition, a clinical trial is always an interventional study, as it evaluates one or more investigational medicinal products (not used in clinical practice, under the conditions in which the study is conducted). However, not all interventional studies are clinical trials of investigational medicinal products. The definition of "clinical intervention study" can be broader:

Any research that advocates a change, influence or scheduling of health care, behavior or knowledge of participants or caregivers, with the aim of discovering or verifying effects on health, including exposure to medicinal products, use of medical devices, performance of surgical techniques, exposure to radiotherapy, application of cosmetic and body hygiene products, physiotherapy intervention, psychotherapy intervention, use of transfusions, cell therapy, participation in individual or group educational sessions, diet intervention, intervention in access to or organization of health care or intervention designated as unconventional therapy.

Figure 7 - Clinical trials and other intervention studies.

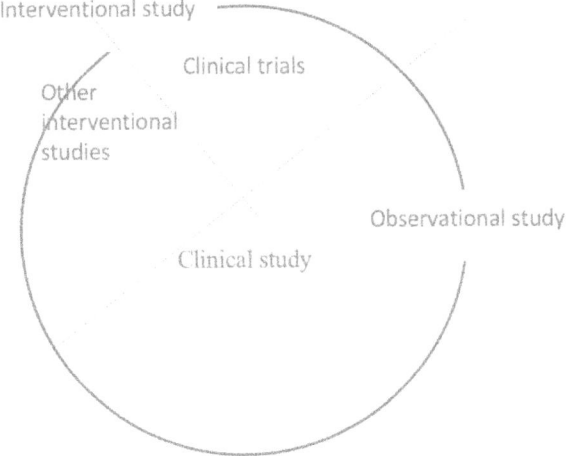

Chapter 16 - Phases of Clinical Trials

Classically, four phases are defined for clinical studies (phase 1, 2, 3 and 4). The phases define the research trajectory that will allow a given medicinal product to obtain a Marketing Authorization if it is approved in them. Successively, phases 1 to 4 involve more people, assuming that the inherent risks are progressively lower for participants as the safety profile of the drug under study becomes better known. At the same time, the main objectives of the studies in each phase differ, starting with the evaluation of the pharmacokinetic and pharmacodynamic profile, drug interactions, dose and therapeutic window, and then focusing more on efficacy. The evaluation of safety, effects and adverse reactions is present throughout the process.

This conventional 1-2-3 phase model has been challenged, considering that there are many situations in which the definition of the phases is not strict and their objectives are mixed. Currently, intermediate designs have emerged, such as phase 1-2 studies. They evaluate people with the disease and not healthy volunteer individuals, which is characteristic of phase 1, but also dose-response and maximum tolerated dose, characteristic of phase 2 (32,33). There are also phase 2-3 studies, which aim to reduce the time needed to evaluate a new molecule, shortening the transition time from phase 2 to confirmatory phase 3 studies (34).

According to FDA estimates, approximately 30% of drugs under evaluation do not pass phase 1, of these, 66% do not pass phase 2, and of these, 75% do not successfully complete phase 3, after which they could receive marketing authorization. In other words, it is estimated that only 5 to 6% of drugs entering Phase 1 testing successfully complete Phase 3 and can be marketed (35). The motto "Fail early and fail fast" has been adopted in the development of new drugs, increasing the importance of phase 1 and 2 studies (36).

Chapter 17 - Phase 1 Clinical Trials

Phase 1 clinical studies are guided by the principle of "safety first". They are the first studies in human beings and are based on information collected from so-called preclinical studies. Translational research on a new drug is based on the assumption that results obtained in the laboratory or in animal models can predict results in humans. However, it is important to note that this predictability can be compromised if the animal models used are not suitable for the mechanism of the disease in question in humans. This is even more relevant when dealing with the first drug of a class with a new mechanism of action (37).

It is important to ensure that the drug has been previously tested in different animal models, with comparable results (clinical effect and safety profile). Consistent results across animal species improve the predictability of its application in humans. Consistency of results is also relevant in defining a therapeutic window. There are different ways to determine the initial dose for a first-in-human study. The most traditional approach is based on the dose that does not produce adverse effects in the most sensitive animal species (the no observable adverse effect level - NOAEL). If the drug is not very toxic, an initial dose based on the NOAEL may already be pharmacologically active (37).

Another approach to estimating the initial dose is based on the minimum anticipated biological effect level (MABEL) (37).

The methods used to estimate the dose in humans based on preclinical data depend not only on the mechanism of action of the drug but also on its pharmacokinetic properties. There are several ways to estimate the human equivalent dose, depending on the different animal species, the drug profile, and the routes of administration. The simplest method is to standardize the dose in mg/kg with a fixed conversion factor for each animal species.

In methodological terms, Phase 1 studies aim to characterize the pharmacokinetic profile - absorption, metabolism, distribution, and elimination of the drug, characterize its pharmacodynamic profile and interactions with food or other drugs, and assess safety and dose (from a safety perspective) (36).

These studies are usually conducted in healthy volunteer subjects, as their main objective is to define the basic pharmacokinetic and pharmacodynamic profile. However, although this remains the norm, several issues have been raised. For drugs whose mechanism of action determines the occurrence of expected but serious adverse effects, such as many antineoplastics, it is not considered ethical to expose healthy volunteers to Phase 1 studies. In these circumstances, Phase 1 studies are conducted in people with the target disease, as it is assumed that they may benefit from exposure to the drug.

The ideal dose of the test drug is determined by several strategies. The most common study design advocates progressive escalation of the dose until toxicity is observed in more than 33% of participants (i.e., 2 out of 6). At this point, the dose escalation should be stopped, and the dose should be reduced to the dose tested just before toxicity was recorded in one-third of people, with this dose being evaluated in a new group of participants. The goal of reevaluating this dose is to try to collect as much data as possible on the dose to be used in future Phase 2 clinical studies (38).

In practice, you can use the so-called 3+3 design. In this type of design, groups of 3 subjects are included at a time. A given dose is administered to all 3 individuals if no dose-limiting toxicity (DLT) is observed. DLT is defined as the occurrence of a clinically significant adverse event or the occurrence of a laboratory value outside the normal range (grade 3 or 4 adverse event), which cannot be attributed to disease progression, intercurrent illness, or other drugs.

If no DLT situations are observed in these three individuals, the dose can be increased to the next level and three more individuals can be included and so on. If two or more DLT situations occur, the escalation should be stopped, and the administered dose is defined as the maximum administered dose (MAD). If this happens at the evaluation of the first 3 persons participating in the study, you must include 3 more people, but they will take a lower dose.

If you find 1 DLT in a group of 3 persons, you should include 3 more persons in the study and if you do not find any DLT, you can increase to the next dose and include 3 more people. If you find 1 or more DLT (in the second group of 3 persons included after the appearance of 1 DLT), you should stop the dose escalation, and the administered dose will be defined as MAD (36).

The maximum dose at which 0 or 1 DLT occurred, after administration to 6 individuals, is considered the maximum tolerable dose (MTD) and is usually recommended for use in phase 2 clinical studies (36).

There are other types of Phase 1 study designs, especially those included in accelerated development programs, for example, in the oncology field. In these designs, the dose titration phase is faster, and dose increases are performed in the same person.

In summary, from the study design point of view, Phase 1 studies are non-comparative studies in which participants are gradually included in an attempt to minimize safety concerns.

Regarding the population, that is, the people included in Phase 1 studies, I have already mentioned that it is not always ethical to include healthy volunteer subjects, given the safety profile of some drugs. A very important issue for the validity of the results of phase 1 studies is that the healthy volunteer subjects included are usually young, male, and white. This selection bias questions the external validity of the results, knowing that in most diseases, people are older and that drugs will be administered to all people, regardless of sex, gender identity, skin color, ancestry, or culture (39).

In 1977, the FDA issued a guidance that excluded "women of childbearing potential" from phase 1 and 2 clinical studies (40). This definition included all women capable of becoming pregnant, regardless of their sexual activity, use of contraceptives, sexual orientation, possible infertility of the partner, or desire to become pregnant. This standard was based on protecting women from the possible teratogenic effects of drugs under development. However, several studies have indicated that this effect can also occur through sperm (41,42).

This ban was in effect until 1993, and many drugs entered the market after a clinical research process in which women were clearly underrepresented (43). In 1993, the FDA revised its position and recommended that clinical trials include both men and women in adequate numbers to allow for the detection of significant differences between the sexes in terms of pharmacological response (44). Despite this guidance, equal participation of women is far from being a reality.

Specifically, with regard to Phase 1 studies, a study published by Pinnow et al. (45) estimates that only 30.6% of the people participating in phase 1 studies are women, and 34.1% of phase 1 studies are exclusively of male participants.

Therefore, there is a clear bias associated not only with gender but also with age, skin color, ancestry, and culture (46). This bias is serious because it has been established that there are differences in physiology, pathophysiology, and patterns of gene expression among people of different ages, between men and women, between people with different gender identities, and from different geographic regions (47). Assuming the above differences, it is to be expected that the pharmacokinetic and pharmacodynamic profile, dose, and safety profile are different according to age, sex, gender identity, ancestry and socio-cultural background, so it is essential that all individuals can be included in clinical studies, from phase 1 onwards (48).

Examples of Phase 1 Studies

The presented studies are real studies and the information was extracted from the clinicaltrials.gov registry. Although the example omits the name of the drug being tested, the associated bibliographic references provide access to the study.

Original title omitting the drug name: A Phase 1, Open-Label, Non-Randomized, 2-Period, Fixed Sequence, Study to Assess the Absolute Bioavailability and Fraction Absorbed of 'drug A' in Healthy Male Subjects (49).

Study Characteristics

- Study Type: Interventional, single-arm, non-comparative.

- Intervention: Drug for the treatment of type 2 diabetes.

- Sample Size: 8 participants.

- Randomization: No.

- Blinding: Open-label.

- Duration: Up to the last follow-up assessment, 27 days.

- Primary Endpoint: Area under the serum concentration-time profile curve, from time zero to the time of last measurable concentration (Dose normalized to 1 mg) - measure of average plasma drug concentration levels after dose administration. Absolute oral bioavailability.

• Secondary Endpoints (examples): Time to peak concentration; elimination half-life; apparent volume of distribution; number of participants who recorded adverse events; number of participants who discontinued the study due to adverse events.

• Eligibility Criteria:

o Inclusion Criteria:

Healthy males aged 18 to 65 years.

Body Mass Index (BMI) of 17.5 to 30.5 kg/m2; and total body weight > 50 kg.

o Exclusion Criteria (only some of the criteria are presented):

Evidence or history of clinically significant hematologic, renal, endocrine, pulmonary, gastrointestinal, cardiovascular, hepatic, psychiatric, neurological, or allergic disease (including drug allergies, but excluding untreated asymptomatic seasonal allergies).

A urine test positive for drugs of abuse or recreational drugs.

Positive results for hepatitis B surface antigen (HBsAg), hepatitis C virus antibody (HCV Ab), or human immunodeficiency virus (HIV).

History of alcohol abuse or excessive alcohol consumption and/or any other use or dependence on illicit drugs.

Current smokers and those who have smoked any substance in the last 12 months.

This is a typical phase 1 study design. It is a study of an antidiabetic drug, administered orally and intravenously, with the objective of characterizing the pharmacokinetic profile and evaluating safety at predetermined doses.

It includes only 8 individuals who are evaluated after ingesting the drug orally and subsequently after intravenous administration.

All tested individuals were male. Their ages ranged from 18 to 65 years and there was no explicit mention of skin color or ancestry in the eligibility criteria. However, the 8 participants included were White and aged between 25 and 55 years.

The eligibility criteria exclude obese individuals with BMI > 30.5 kg/m2, exclude individuals with pathologies of any type, and exclude smokers.

The eligibility criteria should be analyzed to ensure that the biases they impose are not significant enough to compromise external validity. Most people with diabetes are over 55 years of age, many are obese, smokers, and have concomitant diseases and risk factors, and certainly include women and people of any skin color, ancestry or culture. Estimating the pharmacokinetic profile by evaluating only relatively young White men will likely lead to results that cannot be extrapolated to the target population.

Original title omitting the drug name: A Phase 1 Study to Evaluate the Safety, Immunologic and Virologic Responses of 'X Therapy' in HIV-Infected Individuals on Suppressive Antiretroviral Therapy (50).

Study Characteristics

- Study Type: Interventional, sequential with dose escalation.

- Intervention: Drug for HIV-1 (doses of 0.1, 0.3, 1.0, 3.0, 10.0, 30.0, 100.0, 300.0 and multiple doses of 300.0 micrograms/kilogram (μg/kg)).

- Sample Size: 21 participants.

- Randomization: No.

- Blinding: Open-label.

- Duration: Up to 77 days.

- Primary Objective: Number of patients with adverse events and serious adverse events between the first and last study assessment.

- Secondary Objectives (examples): Peak plasma concentration; time to peak concentration; half-life.

- Eligibility Criteria:

o Inclusion Criteria:

Individual's ability and willingness to provide written informed consent.

HIV-1 infection, documented by any approved rapid HIV test (...).

Potent, stable, and continuous ART regimen ≥ 24 months prior to enrollment.

Plasma HIV-1 RNA < 50 copies/mL at two timepoints within the previous 12 months of enrollment and never ≥ 50 copies/mL at two consecutive timepoints within the past 24 months.

Adequate organ function based on acceptable laboratory parameters.

o Exclusion Criteria (only some of the criteria are presented):

Women of childbearing potential, i.e., any woman who has had menses and has not undergone surgical sterilization or menopause.

History or other evidence of severe disease, immunodeficiency other than HIV, (...).

This is a typical study design to determine the dose of a new drug and evaluate its safety profile.

It includes 21 participants, with no reference to sex or gender. However, the exclusion criteria state that "women of childbearing potential, defined as any woman who has had menses and has not undergone surgical sterilization or menopause" cannot participate, which effectively excludes nearly all adult women. In fact, this study ended up including only men.

The biases in the eligibility criteria can be both explicit, as when it is mentioned that only men can participate, and implicit, as in this case.

Chapter 18 - Phase 2 Clinical Trials

Phase 2 studies are designed to evaluate whether the investigational drug has sufficient potential efficacy to justify proceeding to larger Phase 3 clinical studies. At the same time, Phase 2 studies will increase the available safety information and assess the optimal dose, taking into account safety but also the dose-response relationship.

Phase 2 studies are usually controlled and often randomized, and are conducted with a relatively small number of people with the disease being evaluated (from a few dozen to a few hundred).

These studies use the dose previously considered safe, in an attempt to evaluate its tolerability in a larger number of people while simultaneously assessing its efficacy. Thus, the most characteristic objectives of Phase 2 studies are the evaluation of safety, efficacy and dose, seeking to more definitively establish the ideal doses that will then be used in Phase 3 studies. Eligibility criteria are generally restrictive and the included population is very homogeneous.

Sometimes a subdivision into phase 2a and phase 2b studies is used. According to this segmentation, phase 2a is intended for dose evaluation, including small groups of participants who will be administered an increasing dose of the drug, evaluating the dose-response relationship. Phase 2b includes studies aimed at assessing the drug's efficacy in terms of success in treating, preventing or diagnosing a disease.

Phase 2 studies should be designed to minimize the risk of exposure to an ineffective or toxic drug. Therefore, they are usually of short duration or have planned interim analyses over time.

In single-arm studies, the patient group is submitted to the new drug being tested, with no control group. This design is mainly used in oncology or in situations of serious diseases for which there is no effective therapeutic alternative. In these situations, we simply assess the number of patients with therapeutic success and then compare the success rate with that of known alternatives (historical control) or with the clinical expectations of the situation, to decide whether or not to proceed to phase 3.

In comparative studies, which are usually randomized, the design is similar to that used in phase 3 studies. The patient population is randomly assigned to one or another treatment. The patient population is randomly assigned to the experimental drug or to the control group, either another active drug or a placebo. Although similar to phase 3 studies, these studies involve smaller samples and use endpoints that can be assessed in a short period of time.

Another possible design for phase 2 studies are studies where there is no active or placebo comparator, but the enrolled population is randomly assigned to two or more experimental drugs, and the best performing one is selected to continue the research process through additional phase 2 or 3 studies.

Some less conventional designs have been used to reduce the time of the research process without compromising the quality of results.

In this chapter, I describe three designs of what are considered master protocols, that is, single protocols evaluating multiple hypotheses, interventions and/or clinical situations (51): umbrella trials, basket trials and platform trials.

In umbrella studies, several experimental drugs, alone or in combination, are used to treat one disease/situation (called an "umbrella"). For example, patients with lung cancer can be included in a study and subdivided according to the molecular specificities of the tumor (biomarkers) and randomly assigned to different experimental drugs.

"Basket" studies include patients with different types of tumors with the same molecular specificity (same biomarker), who are treated with an experimental drug (the same for all those included).

In either of these designs, one of the study arms can be turned into a randomized controlled "sub-study". In other words, participants with a particular tumor type and biomarker may be randomized to the study drug or a comparator.

The main strength of umbrella studies is their flexibility, which means that when one of the biomarkers is rare, it can still be included in the other arms, allowing new study arms to be added or existing ones to be withdrawn. The main weaknesses are the possibility of delays or very small samples if one of the diseases is rare, or if the biomarker is rare, and also the fact that there is no comparison arm to validate the results.

The main strength of basket studies is the possibility to carry over results from similar studies in other diseases, and they are more efficient than separate studies for each disease, as they use a single protocol and logistics. The main weaknesses are similar to those of umbrella studies.

In comparative terms, patients in umbrella studies have a single disease and can be divided into subgroups based on risk factors, while patients in basket studies have multiple diseases with a common unifying factor (biomarker or risk factor), and the different diseases may form subgroups for analysis. In both types of studies, there may be comparison groups, and in that case randomization may occur. The control may be another active drug or placebo (52).

Platform trials are studies that evaluate multiple interventions against a fixed control group. In this design, adaptive conditions are predefined that allow for the removal of interventions that prove to be ineffective over time and the addition or loosening of others (53).

As I've already mentioned, eligibility criteria for phase 2 studies are often restrictive, leading to the evaluation of very homogeneous populations. Although on one hand this may be justified by the need to increase internal validity given the small number of participants, on the other hand, including very homogeneous individuals compromises the external validity of the results, i.e., their extrapolation to the real population that could benefit from the intervention being assessed.

Examples of phase 2 studies

The studies presented are real studies and the information was extracted from the clinicaltrials.gov registry. Although the name of the drug being tested is omitted in the example, the associated bibliographic reference allows access to the study through the website.

Original title omitting the name of the drug: A Phase 1-2 Study to Assess the Safety and Efficacy of 'drug Y' in Combination With drug A or drug B in Patients With Metastatic Melanoma (54)

Study characteristics

- Study type: Interventional, single-arm, non-comparative.

- Intervention: Drug under evaluation for the treatment of melanoma, used in combination with another drug.

- Sample: 53 participants.

- Randomization: No.

- Blinding: Open label.

- Duration: Up to last follow-up assessment, 12 months.

- Primary endpoint: Objective response rate, using RECIST v1.1 criteria.

- Secondary endpoints (examples): Progression-free survival time; overall survival time; adverse events and serious adverse events.

- Eligibility criteria (examples):

- Inclusion criteria:

o Individuals 18 years of age or older.

Histologically confirmed metastatic melanoma with measurable disease, stage III or stage IVA, IVB or IVC disease.

Symptomatic or radiographic progression while on or after treatment with "drug X" administered as monotherapy or in combination.

Women of childbearing potential and men must agree to use effective contraceptive methods from enrollment, throughout the study treatment period, and for at least 90 days after the last dose.

o Exclusion criteria (only some of the criteria are presented):

>Patients who have received systemic treatment with "drug Z" within 6 months prior to study entry.

>Patients with active autoimmune disease that requires disease-modifying therapy.

Patients with any form of active primary or secondary immunodeficiency.

Patients with active systemic infections requiring antibiotics or active hepatitis A, B, or C.

Patients with known diagnosis of human immunodeficiency virus (HIV) infection.

Women who are pregnant or breastfeeding.

This is a typical phase 2 study design. It is a study of a drug for the treatment of advanced melanoma. It is an open-label study in which the new drug is used in combination with two other drugs already in use. The comparison is made between patients using the new drug in combination with each of the other drugs.

Importantly, the goal of this study is to evaluate the efficacy of the new drug in each of the combinations, through response rate, but also progression-free survival and overall survival. The primary endpoint is the one that can be achieved in the shortest possible time (response rate). Regarding the profile of the participants, analysis of the study results showed that 62% were male and 89% had white skin (54).

Title: A Multicenter Phase 2 Study of the Glutaminase Inhibitor CB-839 in Combination With Paclitaxel in Patients With Advanced Triple Negative Breast Cancer (TNBC) Including Patients of African Ancestry and Non-African Ancestry

Study Characteristics

- Study Type: Interventional, 4-arm, comparative.

o Cohort 1: African ancestry patients who received 2 or more prior lines of therapy for metastatic disease.

o Cohort 2: African ancestry patients who have not received prior therapy for metastatic disease.

o Cohort 3: Same as Cohort 1 but in non-African ancestry patients.

o Cohort 4: Same as Cohort 2 but in non-African ancestry patients.

- Intervention: Investigational drug for the treatment of patients with triple negative breast cancer, used in combination with another drug.

- Sample Size: 52 participants.

- Randomization: No.

- Blinding: Open-label.

- Duration: Up to last follow-up assessment, 12 months.

- Primary Endpoint: Overall response rate, using RECIST v1.1 criteria.

- Secondary Endpoints (examples): Progression-free survival time; overall survival time.

- Eligibility Criteria (examples):

o Inclusion Criteria:

Women 18 years of age or older.

Advanced triple-negative breast cancer.

Participants must self-identify as being of African ancestry (including African American) for inclusion in cohorts 1 and 2.

No prior systemic treatment for advanced or metastatic disease for inclusion in cohorts 2 and 4.

2 or more prior lines of systemic treatment for advanced or metastatic disease, including a taxane, for inclusion in Cohorts 1 and 3.

This study was designed to evaluate the same treatment regimen in women with advanced triple-negative breast cancer who have and have not received prior systemic treatments, subdividing the objectives to specifically evaluate women who self-identify as being of African ancestry and those who do not. This is an example of a study that aims to provide specific evidence for a minority/vulnerable group. This type of study specifically targeting minority/vulnerable groups, for common diseases that affect everyone, is a very important step towards equality and inclusion in health in general. It should be noted that this study does not merely conduct subgroup statistical analyses, nor are these subgroups targets of the study.

Chapter 19 - Phase 3 Clinical Trials

Phase 3 studies are designed to evaluate the efficacy of a therapeutic intervention in larger samples and over a longer period of time than those used in Phase 2 studies.

Phase 3 studies are comparative studies that evaluate the outcomes of the intervention being studied compared to other known interventions or placebo. Whenever possible, they are randomized and blinded. The number of people included can range from tens to thousands.

Randomization

Randomization is a method used to randomly and unpredictably divide the people participating in a clinical study into different study arms (groups). An arm or group is each of the therapies being tested, whether it is the one motivating the study or those used as comparators. Thus, a two-arm study is one in which an intervention under evaluation is compared to a single comparator, which may be another active therapy or a placebo, if there is no therapy of proven efficacy in the indication being evaluated. A three-arm study has one group that will undergo the experimental intervention and two groups that will be controls, or vice versa. The distribution of participants among the different study arms can be equal, i.e., have the same number of patients in each arm (described as 1:1 if the study has two arms or 1:1:1 if the study has three arms, and so on), but it can also be asymmetric, with more people in the experimental arm than in the comparison arm, for example, 2:1, which means there will be two people included in the experimental arm for every one person included in the control arm. The main rationale for an asymmetric distribution is the inherent risk-benefit assessment of the drugs or interventions in question. Randomization by generation of random numbers (performed by computer systems) allows people to be allocated among the study arms randomly and unpredictably, i.e., the fact that one person goes to one group does not predict where the next person will go.

In the case of a simple randomization and an equal ratio between two groups (1:1), half of the people will be randomly assigned to intervention A and half to intervention B, but it may happen that when 300 people are included, the first 100 people will remain in group A. This will not be a problem if the study is conducted randomly. This will not be a problem if the study includes the entire intended sample and all individuals complete the stipulated evaluation periods, but if the study is interrupted early or for some reason does not include all 300 individuals, the results will be affected by the possibility that the first individuals are all in group A.

Block randomization avoids this type of distribution. In the example above, if block randomization had been used, participants would have been randomly assigned to intervention A and intervention B, half to each, but in groups (blocks). Blocks should always be greater than 2, multiples of the number of interventions (in this case, multiples of 2), and divisors of the total sample (in this case, 300). If we consider blocks of 6, we would have 50 blocks for this study, in which there would always be 3 people randomized to intervention A and 3 people randomized to intervention B.

Randomization allows avoiding selection biases inherent to a choice made by researchers or patients. Moreover, randomization allows the characteristics of the participants to be equally distributed among the study arms, i.e., as long as the sample is large enough, the percentage of women in the study arms is likely to be similar, the mean age will be similar, the severity of the disease will be similar, and so on. Randomization allows us to balance between study groups not only the characteristics we know and anticipate may influence the results, but also those we do not know or do not assess.

Stratification

Stratifying a clinical study sample means subdividing people into groups before randomly assigning them to different interventions. For example, people in a given study may be stratified according to the severity of their illness and whether or not they have received previous treatment, before being randomly assigned to the experimental intervention or control. This ensures that there will be the same number of people with severe disease in each study arm and also the same number of people already exposed to other treatments.

Stratification is useful in large samples when one wants to analyze results by subgroups (according to the defined strata) or when one anticipates that the characteristic in question may be a critical factor for response.

Study Designs

In the previous chapter, I presented the "umbrella", "basket", and "platform" designs. In this chapter, I will describe the more classical phase 3 study designs, namely the "parallel" design and the "crossover" design.

In the parallel design, two or more groups of participants are followed (Figure 8). In the case of a randomized study, eligible individuals are randomly assigned to the different study arms (drug(s) under test and control(s)) and followed for the stipulated evaluation period.

In the crossover design, eligible individuals are initially assigned to the study arms, usually two, as in a parallel design study (Figure 9), and in a second phase switch from arm X to arm Y and vice versa. Depending on the intervention, a washout period between the two may be necessary.

Compared to studies with a parallel design, studies with a crossover design have the advantage that people are compared with themselves when exposed to intervention X and intervention Y. Since people are evaluated at two time points, the study sample can be smaller. On the other hand, the study duration will be longer as it consists of two consecutive evaluation periods.

The main limitation of using crossover designs is that they can only be considered when it comes to a disease that is stable over time and whose treatment does not have curative or disease-modifying effects, as in this case people would not be in the same circumstances at the beginning of the second part of the study (after crossover). Crossover designs have been applied in studies, for example, in asthma or migraine prevention, in some studies on type 2 diabetes or hypertension.

Figure 8 - Parallel studies.

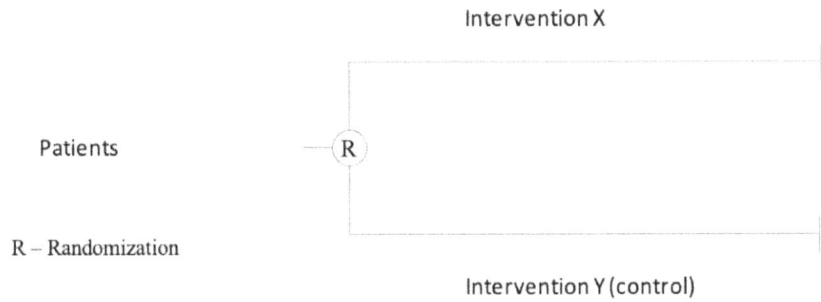

Figure 9 - Crossover studies.

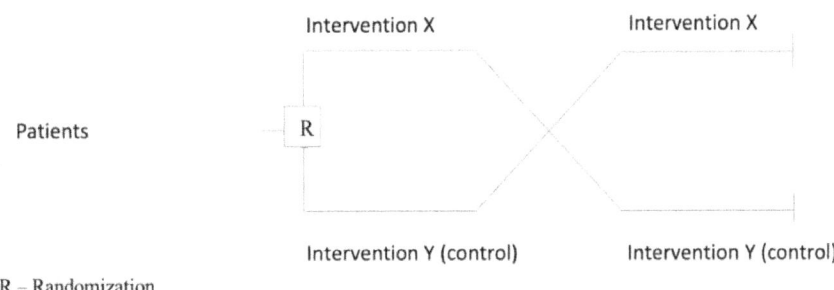

In addition to these designs, there are others that are variations of those already presented, such as:

Sequential design, in which a specific sequence of drugs, administered in different orders, is evaluated;

Factorial design (56), in which individuals can take all interventions simultaneously, only one of them or none of them, and the results are analyzed in all possible combinations, as shown in Figure 10, for a factorial design with two drugs, X and Y, and a placebo, 0.

Figure 10 - Factorial design trials.

		Randomização para tratamento Y	
		Sim (Y)	Não (0)
Randomização para tratamento X			
	Sim (X)	Ambos X e Y (XY)	Só X (X0)	Todos os X (XY e X0)
	Não (0)	Só Y (Y0)	Nem X nem Y (00)	Não X (Y0 e 00)
		Todos os Y (XY e Y0)	Não Y (X0 e 00)	

Another type of design that can be very useful in personalized medicine is the so-called n=1 design. These studies involve a single person who receives an intervention and a control, which can be no intervention or a placebo. If we consider that N is no intervention, P is placebo, and X is the drug being tested, we can have the following types of n=1 studies, whose sequence can be pre-specified or randomized:

- N-X (quasi-experimental design, does not demonstrate association)

- N-P-N (experimental design, evaluation of placebo effect)

- N-X-N (experimental design, drug evaluation)

- N-P-X-P-X-N (experimental design, drug versus placebo evaluation)

If, in an n=1 design in which the person is successively exposed to the drug and control, it is demonstrated that there is improvement during the drug period and no improvement during the placebo or no treatment period, the cause-effect association has been demonstrated.

Population

In Phase 3 studies, the eligibility criteria are generally broader than those we use in Phase 2 studies. In recent years, there has been a trend to make eligibility criteria less restrictive, allowing the inclusion of more diverse individuals, which enables greater external validity of the results and greater clinical applicability. As the heterogeneity of tested individuals increases, studies sometimes have less internal validity because potential confounding factors tend to increase.

The importance of diversity and inclusion in clinical trials

Based on the fact that different people may express, evolve, and react differently to the treatment of the same disease, it is crucial that clinical trials reflect the diversity of real clinical practice.

With respect to clinical trials, some fundamental aspects of human diversity have been factors of exclusion (or lesser inclusion) of certain population groups, and in some situations, the diseases in question are even more prevalent in those same groups. This systematic exclusion has two direct consequences: first, it prevents the benefits of scientific advances from being equitable and transversal, and second, it gives us a false sense of knowledge, not applicable to everyone, which can lead to harmful practices. The main factors that can influence disease risk, health outcomes, and treatment response are (5):

- Age;

- Sex assigned at birth;

- Pregnancy;

- Life experiences (negative, such as psychosocial stress and lack of basic resources, or positive, such as educational and employment opportunities);

- Health-damaging behaviors (e.g., psychoactive substance use, sedentary lifestyle, overeating, risky sexual behavior);

- Healthy behaviors (e.g., adequate sleep, preventive behaviors, physical activity, healthy eating);

- Environmental conditions (e.g., pollution, access to health services or healthy foods, neighborhood segregation);

- Genetic variation and geographic ancestry;

- Underlying medical pathology or presence of comorbidities.

As we have seen, clinical trials have historically favored the inclusion of men, white-skinned individuals, and those under 65 years of age, without taking into account population diversity, disease characteristics, or treatment. This disparity in access has consequences not only for population health but also for scientific knowledge itself.

Based on the fact that older adults are the most affected by diseases, is it appropriate to exclude them from clinical drug trials from which they could benefit? Of course, older adults also have more comorbidities and are likely to be polymedicated, but these factors are part of reality and should not be a reason for exclusion. Furthermore, it is plausible to assume that drug metabolism may be different in older individuals, which is why we should question the extrapolation of pharmacokinetic and pharmacodynamic results obtained in phase 1 studies when conducted exclusively in groups of young men.

Since 1993, the National Institutes of Health has issued several guidelines to provide diversity in the inclusion of study participants, including the NIH Policy and Guidelines on the Inclusion of Women and Minorities as Subjects in Clinical Research (57).

According to a study published in 2018, which evaluated the inclusion of women and individuals from minority groups in 107 NIH-funded clinical trials conducted between 2004 and 2009 in the United States, in diseases that were not sex-specific, the proportion of women was 46%, with women representing less than 30% of participants in 15% of studies and less than 15% in 7% of studies (58).

A study published in 2020 found that, in an analysis of 143 clinical trials (290,000 participants) that led to FDA approval of 35 cardiometabolic drugs between January 2008 and December 2017, women represented only 36% of the participant population (and only 30% in studies conducted in North America), while they represent more than 50% of the population in the United States (59).

In April 2022, the FDA published "Diversity Plans to Improve Enrollment of Participants From Underrepresented Racial and Ethnic Populations in Clinical Trials," a document that aims to establish goals and objectives for the vast majority of individuals included in clinical trials to be non-white, taking into account the underrepresentation of African Americans, Hispanics/Latinos, Native Americans, Asians, and Native Hawaiians in studies conducted in the United States (60,61).

According to data published in 2019 on 230 oncology clinical trials conducted in the United States between 2008 and 2018, the percentage of Black individuals included was 2.9% in 2008 and 3.6% in 2018 (62).

Many studies assess "race," "ethnicity," or nationality as if they were the same thing, which makes extrapolation and interpretation of the results difficult.

As for the inclusion of individuals belonging to sexual minorities, gender minorities, or socioeconomically disadvantaged groups, the vast majority of clinical trials do not even take these variables into account, making it impossible to evaluate them.

Examples of phase 3 studies:

The studies presented are real studies, and the information was extracted from the clinicaltrials.gov registry. Although the example omits the name of the drug being tested, the associated bibliographic reference allows access to the study through the website.

Original title omitting the drug name: Comparative Efficacy of 'Drug T' Versus 'Drug A' on Blood Viscosity in Peripheral Artery Disease (PAD) Patients With Type 2 Diabetes (T2D) (63)

Study Characteristics

- Study type: Interventional, randomized, triple-blind, three-arm crossover design.

- Intervention: "Drug A" + "Drug T" placebo versus "Drug T" + "Drug A" placebo versus "Drug A" + "Drug T".

- Study design: Sequential crossover.

- Sample: 70 participants.

- Randomization: Yes.

- Blinding: Triple-blind (participants, researchers, and treating physician); double-dummy.

- Duration: Up to the last follow-up assessment, 16 weeks.

- Primary objective: Mean change in blood viscosity (baseline vs. week 16).

- Secondary objectives (examples): Mean change in blood pressure; adverse events and serious adverse events.

- - Eligibility criteria (examples):

o Inclusion criteria:

Signed informed consent.

Women or men aged 18 or older.

Type 2 diabetes mellitus.

Symptomatic peripheral artery disease.

o Exclusion Criteria (only some of the criteria are presented):

Type 1 diabetes, or poorly controlled diabetes (...).

Uncontrolled hypertension (...).

NYHA grade III or IV heart failure.

History of severe liver disease (...).

History of intracranial hemorrhage.

Individuals with anemia.

Individuals who have donated blood or received transfusions within 3 months prior to study inclusion.

Women who have not used at least one highly effective contraceptive method for at least one month prior to study initiation, or who are not willing to use such a method during treatment and for an additional 15 weeks after completion of treatment, unless they have been surgically sterilized or are postmenopausal (...).

Pregnant or breastfeeding women or those planning to become pregnant during the study and/or for up to 15 weeks after the end of treatment.

Individuals who, in the opinion of the research team, are unlikely to be available to perform all protocol-required procedures and visits.

History or evidence of other medical conditions that, in the opinion of the research team or the study sponsor, may jeopardize the individual's safety or interfere with the study. Unreliable as a participant, in the opinion of the research team (e.g., alcohol or drug abuse, or psychosis).

This phase 3 study evaluated the efficacy of two medications, separately and in combination, to modify blood viscosity in patients with type 2 diabetes and peripheral artery disease. The study aimed to have inclusive criteria, including 45% women, a mean age of 72 years, 32% Caucasians, and 59% Hispanics (63).

It is important to note that several inclusion criteria are left to the discretion of the research team, allowing people to be excluded based on the argument that they are "not reliable as participants" or "not expected to comply with all assessments." These criteria are not only ambiguous but also promote the exclusion of the most disadvantaged individuals, exacerbating inequalities. At the same time, strict criteria regarding the possibility of conception and pregnancy were stipulated for the inclusion of women, but there were no such criteria for men (possibility of conception during the study and possible effects of the medication on semen).

Chapter 20 - Phase 4 Clinical Trials

Phase 4 studies are studies conducted after a drug has already obtained marketing authorization. These studies usually involve large groups of people and have a long follow-up period. The goal is to evaluate long-term efficacy (or effectiveness) and safety, allowing the detection of rare (< 1:10,000) or infrequent effects. Importantly, these studies are extremely valuable because by including large groups of participants, they encompass (depending on eligibility criteria) people from minority groups and/or with rare diseases.

Although called clinical trials, if we think about it, Phase 4 studies are usually observational studies, evaluating the efficacy and safety of drugs in real-world conditions, and randomized clinical study designs are less common in Phase 4.

Despite what was said above, it's important to note that there are Phase 4 studies whose design is typical of clinical trials, being randomized and blinded. In this case, they mimic Phase 3 trials but use drugs that are already on the market.

Besides their importance in allowing greater diversity in the type of people studied, Phase 4 studies are also very important for identifying rare adverse effects and drug and non-drug interactions. These studies are used as a privileged source of information for pharmacoeconomic studies, which are required for drug reimbursement requests.

The design and specific characteristics of observational studies are described in the following chapters, so an example of a randomized, blinded Phase 4 study is presented below (the study presented is a real study and the information was taken from the clinicaltrials.gov registry):

Original Title: A Multicenter, Randomized, Double-Blind, Parallel Group, 52-Week Comparison of Asthma Control and Measures of Airway Inflammation in Subjects of African Descent Receiving Fluticasone Propionate/Salmeterol 100/50mcg DISKUS® BID or Fluticasone Propionate 100mcg DISKUS® BID Alone (64)

Study Characteristics:

- Study type: Interventional; 2-arm, comparative.

- Intervention: fluticasone propionate/salmeterol vs fluticasone propionate.

- Sample: 479 participants.

- Randomization: yes.

- Blinding: double-blind.

- Duration: 62 weeks.

- Primary endpoint: Rate of asthma exacerbations, per person, per year.

- Secondary endpoints (examples): Percentage of asthma symptom-free days.

- Eligibility criteria (examples):

- Inclusion criteria:

- African-American subjects 12-65 years of age.

- History of asthma for at least 6 months.

- Have been taking a low dose of an inhaled corticosteroid in the month prior to study start.

- Exclusion criteria:

- History of life-threatening asthma.

- Hospitalization for asthma in the 3 months prior to the study.

This Phase 4 clinical trial has a design similar to Phase 3 studies, being randomized and double-blind. Another aspect that deserves attention is the fact that this study was specifically designed to evaluate subjects of African descent, which is fundamental to optimize specific therapeutic strategies in a disease that has a high prevalence in this group.

Chapter 21 - Other Intervention Studies

In terms of methodology, population and study design, there are no major differences between drug clinical trials and intervention studies evaluating non-pharmacological interventions, which can be comparative or non-comparative, randomized or blinded. Of course, there are techniques that may be more difficult to apply in these types of studies, like blinding.

Let's look at some examples of interventional clinical studies that are not drug trials (the studies presented are real studies and the information was extracted from the clinicaltrials.gov registry):

Original Title: Exercise Intervention for Lesbian, Gay, Bisexual, and Transgender (LGBT) Cancer Survivors and Caregivers (65)

Study Characteristics:

- Study type: Interventional; 2-arm, parallel comparison.

- Intervention: Exercise for cancer survivors performed by person and caregiver vs exercise performed by cancer survivor alone.

- Sample: 140 participants.

- Randomization: yes.

- Blinding: open-label.

- Duration: 42 days.

- Primary objective: Evaluate the effectiveness of an exercise program performed by the cancer survivor with the caregiver vs exercises performed by the cancer survivor only.

- Eligibility criteria (examples):

- Inclusion criteria:

- Survivors: To be included in the study, survivor individuals must:

- Have been diagnosed with cancer (any type of cancer except squamous cell and basal cell cancers [skin cancers]) and have completed primary surgery, chemotherapy, and/or radiation therapy (those on ongoing adjuvant treatment are still eligible).

- Identify as lesbian, gay, bisexual, or transgender, or have a same-sex romantic partner.

- Have a caregiver willing to participate in the study (defined as anyone who has provided emotional support or tangible aid during the survivor's cancer experience).

- Be 21 years of age or older.

- Written informed consent.

- Caregivers: Caregiver individuals must:

- Be referred by a cancer survivor.

- Be 21 years of age or older.

- Written informed consent.

- Exclusion criteria:

- Physical limitations (e.g., cardiopulmonary, orthopedic) that preclude participation in a low-to-moderate intensity walking program

- For caregivers, currently undergoing active treatment for neoplastic disease.

This trial has characteristics that deserve your attention. The first important aspect concerns the objectives and the logic of the study itself. This is a study specifically designed to meet the needs of a minority group, which has its own specificities in terms of dealing with the stress of being a cancer survivor, aggravated by the stress resulting from the discrimination and microaggressions associated with being LGBTQIA+.

A second important aspect concerns the study methodology. In the protocol text (65) there is a description of how the participant sample was identified and recruited. It was a complex process that involved several simultaneous strategies, which involved identifying eligible individuals through the oncology service's electronic systems, where it was possible to simultaneously search for "people who completed cancer treatment" or "people who are going through cancer treatment" and "people who identify as LGBT". At the same time, pre-screening was carried out through direct referral by clinical staff from the oncology service.

As this was a difficult recruitment process, the research team opted for a third strategy, which was to directly advertise the study through websites, social media, newspapers, and flyers. Based on this strategy, those selected were asked to nominate others in a strategy called snowball (see below).

Original title: Improving Healthy Lifestyle Behaviors in Midlife Black Women to Lower Heart Disease Risk (66)

Study Characteristics:

- Study type: Interventional; 2-arm, parallel comparison.

- Intervention: B-SWELL: Stress Well-being program for midlife Black women versus WE: Well-being program for midlife Black women.

- Sample: 50 participants.

- Randomization: Yes, block randomization.

- Blinding: Double-blind.

- Duration: 8 weeks.

- Primary outcome: In this study, the objective is defined by the creation of the B-SWELL program itself, and only the hypothesis defines the parameters to be assessed.

- Hypothesis: The hypothesis is based on the assumption that participants in the B-SWELL program (intervention) demonstrate greater self-efficacy to manage life stress compared to the WE group.

- Eligibility criteria (examples):

- Inclusion criteria:

- Women, ages 40-64, who self-identify as Black or African American.

- Proficiency in English.

- Ability to hear and speak well enough to participate in everyday conversations.

- Access to a telephone with messaging service.

- Access to Wi-Fi.

- Willingness to participate in the entire study.

- Exclusion criteria:

- Recent immigration to the US.

- Incarceration or house arrest status.

- Pregnancy.

- Terminal illness (i.e., advanced cancer, terminal condition, kidney failure requiring dialysis).

- History of Alzheimer's, dementia, or severe mental illness (i.e., suicidal ideation, schizophrenia, or untreated major depression).

Although the study's objective is highly relevant, as stress management and support tools should consider the target population's specificities, it is highly unlikely that the inclusion and exclusion criteria defined in this study can truly identify a homogeneous population with specific needs and a distinct cultural context.

It seems that the study's research team assumed that "women aged 40-64 who identify as Black or African American" would likely be socioeconomically disadvantaged, socially disadvantaged, and potentially even incarcerated, since the selection criteria explicitly include "ability to hear and speak well enough to participate in everyday conversations [in English]," "access to a phone with messaging service," "access to Wi-Fi," while simultaneously stating "incarceration or house arrest" as an explicit exclusion criterion. Most clinical studies do not include incarcerated individuals, primarily due to the ethical and legal restrictions involved, but we do not typically see this exclusion criterion.

When designing a specific study for a vulnerable population, which seems to be the case here, it is crucial to carefully consider how the participating individuals will be selected so that, on the one hand, they are the people targeted by the study and not a diverse group with only gender, age, and skin color in common, and on the other hand, the selection criteria are not written in a biased or discriminatory manner.

One final observation on a methodological issue: although the study's general characteristics mention that it is being conducted in a double-blind manner, in reality, according to the protocol's text, it is the team collecting the data and conducting the telephone assessment that is blinded. It is unlikely that studies involving educational programs or behavioral techniques would allow for participant blinding.

Section V - Observational Studies Real-World Data

Chapter 22 - Observational Studies - Concept

Observational clinical studies are studies in which, in a systematic way and according to a research protocol, a certain reality is observed without interfering with it. It can be defined as:

Non-interventional clinical study:

- Medicines are prescribed, or medical devices are used under the conditions established in the marketing authorization or in the conformity assessment procedure, respectively.

- The inclusion of participants in a specific therapeutic strategy is not predetermined by a study protocol but depends on current practice.

• The decision to prescribe the medicine or use a medical device is clearly dissociated from the decision to include or not include the person in the study.

• No other complementary diagnostic or evaluation procedures are applied to the participants, and epidemiological methods are used to analyze the collected data.

Observational studies can have different objectives and, therefore, can be divided into epidemiological studies and clinical and pharmacological studies. The former include studies on diseases and health determinants, risk factors, or prevention, while the latter include studies on the efficacy and safety of medications and therapeutic interventions, studies on complementary means of diagnosis or prognosis.

In terms of methodology, observational studies can be comparative or non-comparative, that is, a single group of people can be studied (in this context, a group of people is called a "cohort"), or several groups can be studied and compared. In terms of time, they can be cross-sectional or longitudinal, and the latter can be prospective or retrospective.

The design of an observational study depends on its specific objectives. Compared to intervention studies, observational studies have lower internal validity but higher external validity. Internal validity is lower because there is less control over the participating individuals, and they are more heterogeneous and diverse, which means that there are more factors involved that can influence the results. On the other hand, their external validity is higher because, by including people with diverse characteristics, they are closer to the population as a whole, that is, the people studied are more similar to the people to whom we will extrapolate the results.

Chapter 23 - Cross-sectional Studies

Cross-sectional studies evaluate data from a population at a specific point in time, like a snapshot. They are used, for example, to estimate specific prevalences, characterize populations, health determinants, or opinions on a certain topic. Cross-sectional studies allow for establishing associations between variables but not causality, as they do not include the time factor.

As cross-sectional studies have the main objective of characterizing a population, one of the critical points is how the sample is defined (see also Chapter 32). There are several strategies for selecting samples, including:

Simple random sampling: each individual in the target population has the same probability of being included in the sample. It is the most representative and reliable form of sampling, but also the most difficult to perform in practice. Within this type of sampling, stratified sampling can also be applied, which consists of defining subgroups (strata) according to certain characteristics (such as geographic region or age) and then randomly sampling each of the defined subgroups.

Systematic sampling: individuals are selected from x to x, from a predefined list or a route of households previously marked on a map of a locality (random route). It is not as reliable as random sampling, but it is also representative and balanced, in addition to being easier to perform.

Convenience sampling: people who demonstrate a willingness to participate are included. It is a quick and simple method but presents significant selection biases that can compromise the extrapolation of the results.

Snowball sampling: people are invited to participate in the study by others who are already participating. It is a method with selection biases but can be useful in situations where the population we want to study is difficult to identify or agree to participate. This type of sampling has been used in some studies specifically aimed at including the LGBTQIA+ population.

Let's look at some examples of cross-sectional observational clinical studies (the studies presented are real studies, and the information was extracted from the clinicaltrials.gov registry):

Original Title: Obstetrics and Gynecology Residents and Experts' Knowledge of, Attitudes Toward, Practice Behaviors, and Self-confidence Levels of Caring for Lesbian, Bisexual, and Transgender (LBT+) Patients in Turkey; A Descriptive-cross Sectional Study

Study Characteristics

- Study Type: Observational; cross-sectional.

- Sample: 189 participants.

- Duration: Not applicable.

- Primary Objective: Knowledge, attitudes, practice behaviors, and self-confidence levels of Obstetrics and Gynecology residents and specialists in treating lesbian, bisexual, and transgender (LGBTQIA+) people.

- Eligibility Criteria (examples):

o Inclusion Criteria:

- Age 18 to 60 years.

- Actively working as an obstetrician and gynecologist in Istanbul/Turkey.

o Exclusion Criteria:

- LGBT people who work as obstetricians and gynecologists in Istanbul/Turkey.

This is a study that can be classified as a medical education study. It evaluates, in a single assessment, the knowledge and practices of a group of healthcare professionals regarding lesbian, bisexual, and transgender women in the context of gynecology and obstetrics.

The topic of the study is particularly relevant, as several studies point to the low level of specific knowledge and the low level of comfort among healthcare professionals when dealing with LGBTQIA+ people (67).

Therefore, obtaining concrete data is essential for implementing policies and programs that can fill this gap. On the other hand, in the specific case of gynecology and obstetrics, it is known that lesbian women avoid going to healthcare professionals because of insecurity and discomfort, which leads, for example, to less prevention and fewer mammograms (68), and, therefore, a higher mortality rate for diseases such as breast cancer (69), which is diagnosed later and at a more advanced stage.

Chapter 24 - Cohort Studies

As we saw above, "cohort" means a group of people, so a cohort study is a study that follows one or more groups of people longitudinally. Cohort studies are longitudinal and can be prospective or retrospective. Classically, cohort studies aim to answer epidemiological questions by assessing the relationship between exposure to a certain factor and the occurrence of an event. However, studies of a clinical nature, especially comparisons between groups of the therapeutic effect of various drugs used in routine clinical practice, can be considered cohort studies.

Cohort studies are particularly useful when the exposure factor is not frequent or when one wants to observe the occurrence of several events simultaneously. If the event to be evaluated is not frequent, this is not the best methodology. In these situations, a case-control study should be considered (see the next chapter).

Figure 11 - Cohort Studies.

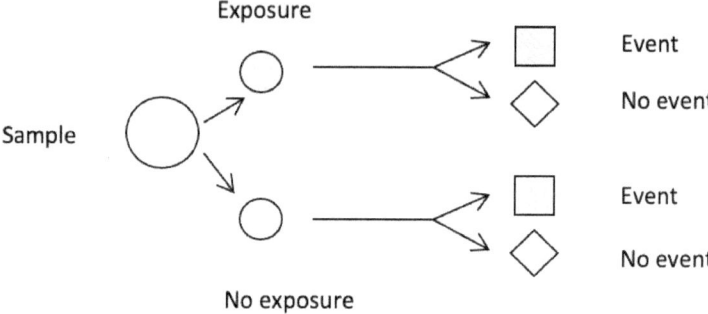

One area where this type of design has been used is in medical education studies, for example, to compare two different training strategies (exposure) and evaluate the outcomes (events).

I would like to draw your attention to the fact that cohort studies can compare more than two groups and can be combined. A matched cohort study is one in which people from one group and another are "matched" based on certain predefined characteristics. The purpose of matching is to reduce possible biases caused by these variables. In simpler terms, it is considered that by having "equal" variables in both groups, these variables no longer have an effect on the results.

When we talk about cohort studies, the Framingham study inevitably comes to mind. The Framingham Heart Study (70) is an epidemiological cohort study that was initiated in 1948 with the objective of assessing the cardiovascular risk of the inhabitants of the city of Framingham, Massachusetts. The study initially included a cohort of 5,209 adults. Participants were evaluated every 3 to 5 years. Currently, this study is analyzing the third generation of participants. It is estimated that more than

3,000 scientific articles have been published based on its results. In general, this study has contributed to increasing the degree of available scientific evidence on cardiovascular risk, confirming associations that we currently consider obvious in our clinical practice, such as smoking is associated with heart disease; increased cholesterol and hypertension are associated with increased cardiovascular risk; physical exercise decreases cardiovascular risk; obesity increases cardiovascular risk; hypertension increases the risk of stroke; in postmenopausal women, the risk of heart disease is higher compared to premenopausal women; psychosocial factors affect the risk of heart disease; high levels of HDL cholesterol are associated with a lower risk of heart disease.

Let's look at other examples of cohort studies (the study presented is a real study and the information was taken from the clinicaltrials.gov registry and a published article):

Original Title: Study of Recently HIV Infected Men and Transmission Behaviors (MetroMates) (71)

Study Characteristics

- Study type: Prospective observational cohort.

- Comparison groups (cohorts): 3 cohorts

    Newly HIV infected men.

    Chronically HIV infected men.

    Men without HIV infection.

- Sample size: 600 men.

- Follow-up period: 12 months.

- Main objective: To compare behavioral patterns of newly HIV-infected individuals to those of chronically infected and uninfected individuals - HIV transmission risks over time.

- Eligibility criteria:

18 years of age or older.

Male.

Documented HIV infection that occurred within the past 12 months.

Willingness to complete study procedures.

Informed consent.

Willingness to refer partners for the study.

Ability to answer questions on the web-based system.

Studies related to HIV infection are often associated with LGBTQIA+ people in a discriminatory way. While there is evidence confirming that the incidence of HIV infection is higher in men who have sex with men (72), there is also evidence showing that women who have sex exclusively with women have a lower incidence of HIV. It is important that when we talk about the inclusion and health specificities of the LGBTQIA+ population, we do not immediately associate them with sexually transmitted diseases.

There are many diseases and risk factors that have different incidences, prevalences, and mortality rates in LGBTQIA+ people.

On the other hand, it is important to have HIV studies that specifically focus on certain minority and/or vulnerable groups, such as men who have sex with men, youth, or women. The disease likely has different characteristics in its progression and control, and optimization of treatment and prevention strategies requires specific knowledge for each group.

Chapter 25 - Case-control studies

Case-control studies are observational studies that compare groups of people based on a particular event (or disease). In other words, the group we call "case" is a group of people who have a certain disease and will be compared to a group of people without that disease, the "control", but who are as similar as possible in terms of control variables, i.e. demographic variables. The objective is to identify if there is an association between the event and exposure to one or more factors.

Due to their characteristics, these studies are retrospective and also have the so-called forward-backward direction, because you identify the event and thus define groups, and then you look back within each group (to the past) and look for exposure to factors that you think may have caused this event.

Case-control studies are particularly useful in situations where events (or diseases) are rare. From a methodological point of view, the main limitation of this type of design is memory bias, which can limit the reliable identification of a given exposure. On the other hand, there is recall asymmetry, i.e., the group of people who had a certain event is more likely to remember having been exposed to a certain factor than the group of people who did not have it.

In these studies, it is possible to establish an association between events and exposures, but it is not possible to draw conclusions about cause and effect.

Figure 12 - Case-control studies.

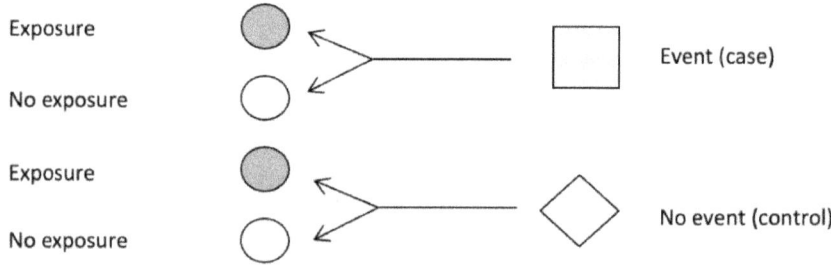

Let's look at some examples of case-control studies (the studies presented are real and the information was taken from the clinicaltrials.gov registry and published articles):

Original Title: Case-control study of risk factors for incident syphilis infection among men who have sex with men in Tokyo, Japan (73)

Study Characteristics

- Study type: Observational, case-control.

- Cases: Eligible persons with evidence of recent syphilis.

- Controls: Persons with characteristics similar to "cases", hospitalized at the same hospital in the same month, with no evidence of recent syphilis.

- Sample: 41 cases, 82 controls.

- Data collection period: Year 2015 (information is analyzed backwards, up to the time recorded in the medical records).

- Main objective: To identify possible risk factors for syphilis, including modifiable behavioral factors.

- Eligibility criteria: Japanese men who self-reported as men who have sex with men (MSM), aged ≥18 years who had had sexual activity (anal and/or oral sex) with another man in the six months prior to study entry.

This study was conducted at a hospital in Tokyo and aimed to analyze the possible risk factors for syphilis, including modifiable behavioral factors. The background of this study is the increase in reports of syphilis in Japan and the need to find personalized and optimized paths for prevention and transmission.

Original Title: Case-Control Study of Renal Cell Cancer Among Caucasians and African Americans in the United States (74)

Study Characteristics

- Study type: Observational, case-control.

- Sample size: 2424.

- Data collection period: Year 2015.

- Main objective: Demographic and clinical characterization of people aged 20 to 79 years with renal cell carcinoma, comparing Caucasian and African American people.

- Eligibility criteria:

    Cases: Residents of study areas diagnosed with histologically confirmed renal cell carcinoma, aged 20 to 79 years, over a four-year period, were eligible for the study.

    Controls: Population-based controls were frequency matched to cases by study site, African-American status, age, and sex in a ratio of one control per case for non-African-American individuals and two controls per case for African-American individuals.

The results of studies like this are important to provide further evidence on health access asymmetries and the harm they cause. This study also allows us to compare cultural, social, and genetic differences in people belonging to minorities or vulnerable groups and analyze their impact on disease, in this case kidney cancer, providing evidence on the subject to enable strategies that promote health equity.

Original Title: A Case Control Study of Women With Multiple Sexual Partners Attending the Jefferson County Department of Health Sexually Transmitted Diseases Clinic (75,76)

Study Characteristics

- Study type: Observational, case-control.

  Cases: Women with 4 or more sexual partners during the previous year.

  Controls: Women with 1 sexual partner during the previous year.

- Sample size: 347 cases; 347 controls.

- Data collection period: Year 2007.

- Main objective: To determine factors that are modifiable predictors of sexually transmitted infection risk in the context of an increase in number of sexual partners by comparing participants with 1 sexual partner to those with 4 or more sexual partners in the past year.

- Eligibility criteria:

- Inclusion criteria:

Female.

Age greater than or equal to 16 years.

Report of 1 sexual partner in previous year or 4 or more sexual partners in previous year.

Written informed consent.

- Exclusion criteria:

Drug and/or alcohol intoxication at time of screening for study.

This study has a case-control design, with retrospective data collection. Considering the objectives, it was to be expected that it would be difficult to collect information from clinical records, i.e., the possibility of assessing risky sexual behavior, alcohol and drug abuse, history of intimate partner violence, depression, and social support, variables described by the research team as part of their objectives. This study was probably only possible because it was conducted at a specific sexually transmitted diseases clinic (Jefferson County Department of Health Sexually Transmitted Disease Clinic, in Birmingham), which may have had the effect of skewing the study toward the user population of that same clinic.

Finally, I must emphasize the importance of the chosen topic, given the discriminatory way in which sexuality in general, and even more so women's sexuality, continues to be addressed.

Section VI - Data collection

Chapter 26 - Data Collection

Data collection is an integral part of all clinical studies. On the one hand, those starting a study tend to immediately think about the questionnaire they will use, but on the other hand, we rarely dedicate the necessary time to analyze how we are writing the questions and response options. Therefore, I will start with two pieces of advice: don't think about the questionnaire until you have defined the protocol well, that is, the objectives and endpoints, and secondly, when working on the questionnaire, think about the type of language you are using and whether the response options for each question are inclusive and reflect diversity.

In clinical studies, we usually collect information through questionnaires and scales, which can be directed to the research team or directly to the people participating in the study, and can be in paper or digital format.

Although the presentation format of the questionnaire may not seem of great importance, there are some practical aspects to consider. Questionnaires in digital format have great advantages over paper:

- They do not involve the manual transfer of information to a database, as the database is created as the person enters the information on the screen, minimizing the possibility of error;

- They allow validation and verification criteria to be run in advance, which also minimizes the possibility of error;

- They allow control over who enters, modifies, or deletes data, and information can be tracked through user and date logging (audit trail);

- They allow a more user-friendly and intuitive presentation, allowing the research team or the person filling in the data to navigate between screens, use multiple options, make options appear or disappear based on previous choices, and consult instructions;

- In longitudinal studies, where each person has multiple data collection moments, they facilitate the combination of information;

- They allow for better levels of data security and protection, as it is possible to define users, passwords, and different levels of access to information;

- They allow for automatic report generation and data analysis.

Despite the increasing use of digital platforms, paper questionnaires still have their place. If you are not a programmer or an experienced user of data collection tools, it is easier to create a paper questionnaire than a digital format one. On the other hand, if it is a scale or a questionnaire to be filled out directly by the participants, for example, a diary to record symptoms or medications, paper is more convenient and often the only option.

When creating a questionnaire, you should ensure that, whenever possible, the questions are closed-ended, presenting the response options in multiple-choice format, except in the case of a question where the answer is a number, for example, age or an analytical value. In these cases, you should collect the number and then transform it into categories. If you directly request the information in the form of a category, you can never go back, that is, if you decide you want another type of division, it will no longer be possible because you don't have the original value. In practice, it is no more work for the person filling out the questionnaire to write a number than to check a multiple-choice option.

Especially in paper questionnaires, it is important to properly mark the response spaces with squares or dashes to facilitate reading and data entry into a database. Avoid leaving open spaces where each person can write freely. For example, if you want a date to be filled in, mark the spaces for the year, month, and day, clearly indicating what corresponds to what.

When creating a questionnaire, we often need to categorize attitudes, perceptions, or opinions, which can be done by defining degrees of agreement. One of the best ways to develop these questions is by using Likert scales.

Likert scales are structured assessments that allow categorizing attitudes, perceptions, or opinions. These scales take the form of graded categories, such as "strongly disagree" to "strongly agree" or "always" to "never". The number of categories varies, with the most common being between 4 and 7. The more categories there are in between, the more difficult the response will be. Scales can have an even or odd number of options. If the number is even, responses can be classified in a binary way as agree/disagree. In scales with an odd number of response options, the "middle" option corresponds to indifference or neutrality. When constructing this type of scale, think about the question you are asking, the objectives of the analysis, and the type of population to which it will be applied.

In the planning phase of your questionnaire, you should organize the questions into groups that make sense to the people who will be answering the questionnaire. If you have questions that you consider more sensitive, present them at the end of the questionnaire.

What type of information is usually collected in a clinical study? Of course, the definition of the data we need depends on the study and its objectives, but there are some variables that are cross-cutting, such as:

> • Demographic or sociodemographic information: they are part of almost all surveys and can be a delicate topic, as they may include questions/answers about sex, gender identity, physiognomic features, geographic origin or ancestry, occupation, income, sexual orientation, or religion. Think carefully about what exactly you want with each of these questions. We will address this in more detail in the next chapter.

• Clinical information: carefully consider who or what can give a reliable answer to what you want to know, i.e., should the variable be answered by the person themselves, by the clinical staff, or by a complementary diagnostic test. For example, if you ask a person participating in your study if they felt nauseous in the last week, you are absolutely right, as the person themselves will be in the best position to answer that question. However, if the question is whether they have atrial fibrillation, the person themselves is probably not the most reliable source of information, and it would be preferable to obtain this information from a medical history (in this case, based on the interpretation of a complementary means of diagnosis).

• Patient-Reported Outcomes: whenever there is a need to collect information about events that occur over time, a diary completed by the participants should be considered (this type of data is called PRO - Patient-Reported Outcomes). There is a memory bias that makes it difficult to collect certain types of information. For example, the recording of adverse events, medication intake, and even satisfaction or quality of life records work better if they are made by the individual in real-time, rather than being requested by the research team at the point of contact.

• Imaging tests: When you need to collect information about imaging tests, think carefully about the quantitative or qualitative parameters that will be recorded, as we usually do not directly analyze images or other records, such as electrocardiogram tracings, which are transformed into numbers and/or classifications.

• Scales: the use of validated scales, whether they are diagnostic, prognostic, response assessment, quality of life, or other scales, is very common and very useful in clinical studies. Validated scales cannot be modified and must be used exactly as recommended by the authors. Before considering using a scale, check if it has been validated for the country and language in which it will be used. Another important aspect is to find out if the scale has royalty payments associated with it.

• Visual analog scales (VAS) are commonly used to assess pain. It is a straight line of 10 centimeters where the left end corresponds to the absence of pain and the right end to the maximum pain that can be imagined. The person is asked to draw a line on the straight line indicating their level of pain. This scale can be used as a straight line or as a line segment with dashes indicating the beginning and end. The same type of scale can be adapted to 0 to 10-point numeric rating scales, or to scales with faces or "emoji" with smiles or tears, mainly used for children. There are also pain scales validated for newborns.

• To assess quality of life, there are several scales, some generic, others for use in specific pathologies. Among the most used are the EQ-5D (30) and the SF-36 (77).

In general, questionnaires should be as short as possible, without any question whose answer is not essential for at least one of the study objectives.

If the study has several assessment points for the same person, this should be clearly reflected in the questionnaire. The end date should always be present.

When designing a retrospective study, it is first necessary to assess what data already exists, as only the information that has been recorded, for example, in a person's clinical file, can be collected.

In general, questionnaires in clinical studies are anonymous and do not allow identifying the person who answered them. In some situations, they have a code that allows identifying the person, but this code has protected and restricted access and is destroyed at the end of the study, being present only to safeguard security aspects, for example, in studies with experimental drugs. No question on the data collection questionnaire should allow direct or presumed identification of the subject.

Chapter 27 - Inclusive Language in Data Collection Instruments

In addition to the technical and scientific issues I mentioned in the previous chapter, one of the most important aspects when creating a data collection questionnaire is the language used.

Questionnaires, like all documents in a clinical study and, more sensitively, all documents that will be read and filled out by study participants, should use gender-neutral language (see Chapter 2). In addition to gender-neutral language, it's important to think about other aspects. Let's revisit the demographic or sociodemographic questions we mentioned earlier. Before you continue reading, I'd like you to think about what questions should be part of the demographic characterization in any clinical study.

Again, the answer should be: it depends on the study objectives. There is no set of questions that must always be part of the characterization. However, there are some questions that appear in almost all studies, so let's examine them one by one.

Age: Age assessment is almost always important to characterize the population participating in a clinical study. It should be asked in years and recorded in numbers, which can be transformed into a categorical scale if needed. Date of birth should not be asked, as it is an element that can lead to identification of the person. If relevant to the research objectives, birth year, or year and month, can be asked.

Sex: When we simply see "sex", we should assume that what is being asked refers to sex assigned at birth. In this case, you should consider the options female, male, intersex. You may consider including the option "I do not want to answer" or "I prefer not to answer". The use of the "other" option should be avoided.

It is very common for questions to arise about whether people in a clinical study should be characterized using sex assigned at birth or their gender identity. Again, it depends. It depends on what you want to assess, but you cannot confuse the two or think they are synonymous (see Chapter 2). If you want to characterize based on anatomical, genetic, or hormonal aspects, then the variable that best fits is probably sex assigned at birth. If your goal is to characterize behavioral aspects and social roles or risk factors, then gender identity should be the chosen variable.

Gender Identity: One should not simply use "gender", because the question you want to answer is what gender the person identifies with. When you ask what the gender identity is, the response options are multiple and difficult to define, as we consider gender identity to be a spectrum. From a practical standpoint, I suggest using a simple, inclusive, and non-discriminatory classification, for example, considering "female", "male", "non-binary" and, in the latter case, "specify" as response options, which will allow you to further categorize the responses. There should be an option that says "I do not want to answer" and another that says "I do not identify with any of the options presented".

It is justifiable to ask about sex assigned at birth and gender identity at the same time if you are conducting a study with specific characteristics in this area. At the same time, it is important to keep in mind that by not systematically asking about gender identity in clinical studies, we prevent segmented analyses that answer specific questions and particularities related to different gender identities.

If you ask whether the person identifies as cisgender or transgender, provide a brief explanation of what you are asking, as many people are not familiar with these concepts.

Marital Status: The question about marital status is simple, as it has a well-defined classification. In this case, you should ask (in gender-neutral language, using the word "person" or "individual" and making the respective gender conjugation) if the person is "single", "married or cohabiting", "divorced or separated", or "widowed". The main issue here is whether marital status provides relevant information for your study. If what you want to know is family context, support network, or whether the person is in an intimate or marital relationship, marital status will not give you that information. It is essential that you find a way to ask exactly what you want to know, even if it is more difficult to formulate the necessary question(s).

Geographic origin or ancestry: We have already discussed in detail the issue of using the term "race" or "ethnicity". The word race is not appropriate when talking about people, and the word ethnicity should be reserved for questions that seek to define whether a person identifies with a group that shares the same culture, history, language, society or nation.

Again, think about what you really want to know. Do you want to know skin color? This makes sense if you're thinking about a study related to, for example, sun exposure or risk of skin cancer, but it won't make sense if you want to measure a social, economic, genetic or epidemiological context, because skin color itself doesn't answer any of those questions. If the goal is to find out a person's origin, then that's the question to ask. The question to ask is not about nationality, as that is a legal issue and also does not provide the desired information, but about place of birth and residence. Place of birth alone is also not enough, as being born somewhere does not imply having lived there (cultural and social heritage), nor does it imply that in terms of ancestry (genetic heritage) the origin is the same. This is one of the most complex questions to get the answers you are looking for and needs to be broken down into several questions that include not only place of birth, but also place of birth of ancestors (or family), as well as the place/country where the person has lived for the longest period of their life. To answer questions related to epidemiological patterns, it may be useful to ask about travel abroad.

Despite the complexity of what I just described, there are still many aspects that are not addressed, for example, we never know if a person who was born in one country and has lived in another since childhood has acculturated to the latter or maintains the habits of the country of origin, which can mean a completely different risk factor profile.

Parenthood and family history: Questions about children should take into account the possibility of them being biological and/or adopted, and this should be explicitly mentioned in the questionnaire. The question should always be formulated in an inclusive way, unless there are objectives that refer to the biological part and, in this case, the question can be divided into two. Questions about pregnancy should not be directly linked to questions about daughters and sons, as this is not inclusive when it comes to adoption situations. More importantly, all questions should be very explicit about what is being considered, making this clear to respondents.

Regarding family history, and assuming that the questions are primarily directed at hereditary situations, refer to "parentage" and not to "mother" or "father".

Sexual Orientation: When asking about a person's sexual orientation, response options should include, in alphabetical order, the following: asexual, bisexual, heterosexual, homosexual (gay or lesbian), pansexual. You should consider the options "I do not want to answer" and "I do not identify with any of the options presented".

Income: If you are asking about income, carefully define the monthly or annual income ranges, explain whether it is individual or family income. In the latter case, you should know how the family is composed.

Religiosity: Questions about religion may be important in some clinical studies. In these cases, instead of knowing about religion, it may be helpful to ask how important religion is in the person's daily life (you can use a Likert scale).

In general, don't forget to present the option "I don't know" if it applies, although you should not do this across the board. Alternatively, you should consider the option "I don't want to answer" or "I prefer not to answer" for questions that everyone is assumed to know how to answer, even if they would prefer not to.

Section VII - Data and Results

Chapter 28 - Variables

In the previous chapters, we looked at some aspects of how to collect data and the type of information that is part of a questionnaire for a clinical study. In this chapter, I propose to take a look at how the data is analyzed.

Think of the study as a whole, as if there were a continuum linking the objectives to the endpoints, the endpoints to the variables, and the variables to the statistical analysis. This continuum reflects the coherence of what you are trying to assess. Let's review some of the concepts I presented above:

- In the objectives, you defined what you want to know.

- In the endpoints, you explained how each of the objectives will be measured.

- Variables translate how you will collect the information that will allow you to determine the endpoints, sometimes directly, meaning the variable reflects the endpoint itself, sometimes indirectly, which requires several direct or calculated variables to determine an endpoint.

The statistical analysis depends on everything we've already said. It depends on the objective - for example, studies aimed at describing, comparing, or associating will require the use of different analysis techniques. But it also depends on the variables being analyzed and how they behave, meaning the type of responses you will get.

Given the importance of defining each variable, it is common to dedicate a few pages of the protocol to characterizing them.

Variables should be described by their name, the units in which they are measured, their description if needed, and their classification (categorical, ordinal, or continuous numeric).

Categorical variables are those that, as the name suggests, represent categories. If there are only two categories, for example a variable whose possible answers are "yes" and "no", it is called a binary variable.

Categorical variables are not ordered, meaning the categories are of equal importance and one is not greater than the other.

Ordinal variables are also variables defined in categories, but these categories have a defined order. In clinical studies, it is common to find examples of ordinal variables when scales are used. For example, imagine a scale from 0 to 7, where you can only get scores corresponding to 0, 1, 2, 3, 4, 5, 6, and 7. This scale is numerical, but it is not continuous because there is nothing between each two numbers; it is not possible to get a score of 5.22 or 6.5.

Another situation where you will find ordinal variables is when you transform continuous numeric variables into classes. For example, imagine a study in which you collected information on age in years. This is a continuous numeric variable, but if you transform this variable into age classes, 0-14; 15-29; 30-49; 50-59; 60-69; ≥70 years, you will have a new variable, now ordinal.

Finally, continuous numeric variables. We call continuous numeric variables those that are measured in numbers and for which we can say that between each two consecutive numbers there are an infinite number of values. For example, laboratory tests such as hemoglobin or cholesterol are continuous numeric variables, as are age or a score on a visual analog scale measured on a straight line in millimeters. If this visual analog scale is scored in numbers with fixed response options from 0 to 10, then the variable is, as we saw before, ordinal.

Continuing with the topic of continuous numeric and ordinal variables, you must keep in mind that you can do calculations with continuous numeric variables, such as differences between values or percentage variation, but you cannot do the same with ordinal variables.

In the next chapter, we will see how the type of variable affects the choice of statistical techniques.

Chapter 29 - Statistical Analysis - General Aspects

In clinical studies, you should define in the protocol the type of statistical analysis that will be performed. In clinical trials and more complex studies, it is common to develop, in addition to the protocol, a Statistical Analysis Plan (SAP) that describes everything that will be done to analyze the data.

In the next pages, I would like to invite you to reflect with me on how we organize the description of the statistical analysis in a protocol. There are several ways to do this, so the one I'm going to give you is just an example.

When describing the statistical analysis, you should include the following points:

- Which population(s) you are going to analyze in relation to which objectives.

- The level of significance you will assume for the statistical analysis.

- Whether the hypothesis is two-tailed or one-tailed (whether one-tailed or two-tailed tests will be used).

- How you will handle missing values.

- How you will describe the variables.

- What statistical techniques (tests) you will apply to answer each objective.

You can also choose to describe how the results will be presented. In this case, you should give examples of the tables (Mock-up Tables) that will be constructed and the type of chart you plan to present.

Population

In a clinical study, it is enough to include in the statistical analysis the information available on all the people who participated. In this case, it is not necessary to define the analyzed population, we simply say that data from all participants will be analyzed.

In clinical trials, it is common to define specific populations, namely those that will be part of the intention-to-treat (ITT) and per-protocol (PP) analyses.

In the ITT analysis, we include all the people who were randomized to a given study group, or all the people who took at least one dose of the drug after being randomized, depending on the study. In the PP analysis, we include only the people who completed the study, meeting the protocol specifications.

What is the big difference between these two analyses? Let's think a bit more in detail about what the main differences are.

In the population considered for the ITT analysis, people who did not complete the study will be considered failures (in relation to what we are measuring in the efficacy objectives), because they have no data. It is true that most people who do not complete a clinical trial drop out due to lack of efficacy or safety concerns, so the assumption that the treatment would not be effective may not be totally wrong. But there are some people who drop out of studies for reasons that have nothing to do with the study or the treatment itself, for example they move homes or they don't like the procedures and simply decide to stop. In these cases, the assumption that the treatment was not effective may not be true. In summary, when, in an ITT analysis, we assume that all people who drop out of the study are failures, we are accepting an "overly" conservative result or, in other words, we are analyzing the results from a more negative perspective.

In the population considered in the PP analysis, we include only the people who completed the study, meeting the protocol specifications, that is, if in a study with two arms (drug A vs control) 100 people were randomly allocated to each arm, but only 80 from each arm completed the study, the ITT analysis includes the 100 people from each arm and the PP analysis includes the 80 who made it to the end. Consider that in the drug A arm 60 people were successful and in the control arm 50 people were successful. The percentage of successes in each treatment will be calculated as follows:

> ITT analysis: successes in drug A group = 60/100, i.e. 60%; successes in control group 50/100, i.e. 50%. Difference between drug A group and control group = 10%.

> PP analysis: successes in drug A group = 60/80, i.e. 75%; successes in control group 50/80, i.e. 62.5%. Difference between drug A group and control group = 12.5%.

In summary, when we assume, in a PP analysis, only the results of the people who completed the study, adhering to the protocol, we are accepting an "overly" optimistic result, because these people will likely be the ones who best tolerated the drug and had the best efficacy results.

In clinical trials we can also consider a population for the so-called "safety analysis", which includes all the people who gave informed consent to participate, even if they were not randomized and did not take any drug for any reason.

It is common to see clinical trials where the research team presents the results for the different populations, which is very useful so we can interpret the meaning of the results obtained.

Keep in mind that the closer the efficacy results obtained by analyzing the ITT and PP population, the more confidence we will have that they are indeed the expected efficacy. Studies where there are many dropouts show greater differences in the results obtained when analyzing the ITT and PP population.

Level of Significance

Formally, the level of significance (or type I error or α error) represents the probability of rejecting the null hypothesis when it is true.

Let's see what this means in practical terms, going back to the clinical study comparing drug A with a control. In this case, the goal is to find out if drug A is more effective than the control, and we agree to measure this efficacy by determining the number of successes in one group versus the other. In this hypothesis, the null hypothesis (called H0) is that there is no difference between drug A and the control (they have similar success rates), and the alternative hypothesis (H1) is that there is a difference between drug A and the control (they have different success rates). When you accept an α error of, say, 0.05, what you are saying is that if the study results (obtained from statistical tests) show that there is a difference between drug A and the control, you will accept those results as statistically significant if the p-value (derived from the applied statistical test) is less than 0.05 (5%). In fact, what you are saying is that you accept as significant the results for which the probability that the difference in the study is due to chance (p-value) is less than the α error level (significance) you set.

Significance values are defined for each study by the research team, with 0.05 or 0.01 being the most commonly used.

In the case of studies that perform multiple comparisons or planned post hoc statistical analyses, significance values should be reduced, minimizing the probability of error.

Study Power

Study power is a statistical concept that refers to the ability of a study to detect a true difference or association, if one exists. In other words, study power is the probability of a study accepting the alternative hypothesis when it is true.

When we talk about study power, we must talk about type II error or β (beta) error. The β error is the probability of accepting the null hypothesis when it is false.

In practical terms, study power is calculated as 1 - β error.

There is no defined value for study power that you should consider, but in most cases it ranges from 80% to 90%.

One-sided or two-sided hypotheses (one-tailed or two-tailed tests)

I would like to use the example above to address another issue. When I defined the hypothesis for our study, I did it as follows:

H0: Outcome (success) of drug A = Outcome (success) of control.

H1: Outcome (success) of drug A ≠ Outcome (success) of control.

This means that the aim of the study is to test whether the outcome of drug A is different from the outcome of the control group, without assuming a priori whether this difference is better or worse. But in some cases this does not make much sense; for example, in a study where we compare a drug with a placebo, it makes more sense to test only if the drug is better than the placebo. In this case, you should state your hypothesis as follows:

H0: Outcome (success) of drug A ≤ Outcome (success) of placebo.

H1: Outcome (success) of drug A > Outcome (success) of placebo.

In terms of choosing statistical tests, these two ways of defining the hypothesis directly influence the choice to perform a given test with two tails (two-tailed test) or with one tail (one-tailed test). One-tailed tests are used when the hypothesis defines a single direction for the effect.

Missing Values

In many studies, the choice is simply not to handle missing values. This means that if there is no response to a given variable for one or more individuals, their values will not be taken into account, and the n (number of people) for that variable will be adjusted according to the actual number of responses. In this situation, n should be clearly shown in all analyses, including in tables and graphs.

If you decide to deal with missing values, you can impute the data, that is, replace the missing data with other data estimated using a specific method, such as imputation using the mean, median, or predictive models. For time series data, missing values can be estimated using interpolation methods, such as linear regression, estimating the missing points from the existing ones.

Chapter 30 - Statistical Analysis - Descriptive Analyses

The description of variables is part of the analysis of all clinical studies. Descriptive analysis includes determining frequencies or values that summarize distributions, such as measures of central tendency (mean and median) and measures of dispersion (standard deviation, interquartile range, maximum and minimum).

Sometimes, when comparing groups and it is important to assess whether the initial overall characteristics are balanced (especially in cases where there was no randomization), the analysis of descriptive characteristics may involve comparing the groups from the beginning. In this case, you should proceed in the same way as in any other comparative analysis (see details below).

For the description of variables, you can consider the following:

- Categorical variables are described by their absolute frequency (n; number of cases) and relative frequency (usually in percentages).

- Continuous numerical variables are described by the mean and standard deviation if the distribution is normal (symmetric or Gaussian distribution) and/or by the median and interquartile range if the distribution is non-normal. The median and interquartile range can also be used for variables with a normal distribution, in which case the median value is similar to the mean value. In addition to the described parameters, the maximum and minimum values found should be presented.

- Ordinal variables can be described in the same way as categorical variables, using absolute and relative frequencies, but they can also be described using the median.

Confidence Intervals

Confidence intervals can be applied to a frequency or to a mean or median value. When you estimate the frequency of a certain event or the mean of a certain variable, you are doing so for the data you collected in the sample. For example, in the sample of 500 people you included in a study, you found that 100 had sleep problems. If you are characterizing the situation in the context of describing the sample, you can conclude that 100 people, 20% of the people studied, had sleep problems. This estimate is accurate, it is a point estimate. However, the purpose of most clinical studies is not to characterize the sample, but to extrapolate the results obtained in the studied sample to the entire population (with similar characteristics). When we make this extrapolation, estimating results for a population from what was obtained in a small group, we are assuming a probability that the value of this estimate is within a certain interval, with a certain margin of error (or, conversely, a certain margin of confidence). If we calculate the 95% confidence interval to estimate the percentage of people in the entire population with sleep problems, we will obtain an interval between [16.5% and 23.5%].

What does this mean? It means that we have a 95% chance of being right if we say that between 16.5% and 23.5% of people in that population have sleep problems. In other words, the probability that there are less than 16.5% of people in that population with sleep problems is 2.5% (half of the estimation error) and the probability that there are more than 23.5% of people with sleep problems is less than 2.5%.

The confidence interval will be 95% if we work on a study with a significance level of 0.05, but it will be 99% if we work on a study with a significance level of 0.01.

The same applies to values obtained from continuous variables and, if the objective is, for example, to extrapolate the mean of a certain variable to the population, you should present the confidence interval for the mean, in addition to the point values for the mean and standard deviation.

Chapter 31 - Statistical Analysis – Comparisons and Associations

Why do we use statistical tests in clinical studies? Statistical tests allow us to estimate the probability that the differences between groups or associations between variables that we find in our sample are due to chance alone, meaning they are not "real". Statistical tests, which can be easily performed with statistical analysis software, allow us to estimate this probability, which is translated into the p-value.

There are many statistical tests, and the choice of which one to use in your analysis depends on your objectives, hypotheses, and variables. In the protocol and the statistical analysis plan, if there is one, you should define the type of test you will use for each objective individually.

Although this is not a statistics manual, I will attempt to describe in a very simple way some of the most common statistical tests in the context of clinical studies. Note that there are many useful tests that will not be described here.

Comparisons between Groups

Before examining the names of the tests or how to interpret the results, let's try to group the characteristics that lead to the choice of one test or another when the objective is to compare groups. Let's start by examining what we call groups and what types of comparisons we might want to make:

- Compare frequencies of a binary categorical variable between 2 independent groups - Compare the percentage (frequency) of success (binary variable) between a group taking drug A and a group taking drug B (2 independent groups), for the treatment of hypertension.

- Compare frequencies of a categorical variable among more than 2 independent groups - Compare the frequency of obesity among adults with female, male, or non-binary gender identity (more than 2 independent groups).

- Compare mean values of a continuous variable between 2 independent groups - Compare mean cholesterol values between people with diabetes who have been treated with oral antidiabetic drugs for more and less than 2 years.

- Compare mean values of an ordinal variable between 2 independent groups - Compare the mean scores on a pain scale used

2 hours after taking a drug are different in those who took drug A or B.

- Compare mean values of a continuous variable between 2 dependent (paired) groups - Comparison of mean cholesterol values in the same group of people before and 6 months after (2 paired groups) a diet and exercise program.

We can summarize the different examples presented taking into account: whether we are comparing 2 groups or more than 2 groups; whether the groups are independent or dependent (paired), i.e., whether it is the same group evaluated at different times, or a case-control study, or any study in which people belonging to different groups have been matched a priori; and whether we want to compare a categorical, continuous numerical, or ordinal variable. Finally, we must evaluate whether, in the case of continuous variables, their distribution is normal or non-normal.

The analysis of the figure below systematizes the type of test applied to each comparison.

Association between variables (choice of tests)

To evaluate whether there is statistical significance in the association between variables, it is first necessary to characterize the variables you are studying. For example, you want to check if there is an association between serum vitamin D and a bone density parameter in a given population. If you are dealing with two continuous numerical variables, the next step is to determine whether the distribution of each of the variables is normally distributed or not, from which it is possible to choose the correlation analysis to be applied, Pearson's correlation or Spearman's correlation.

The correlation values, presented as "r", range between -1 and 1, where values close to 0 mean that there is no association between the variables, values close to 1 mean that when one variable increases, the other also increases or when one variable decreases, the other also decreases, and values close to -1 mean that when one variable increases, the other decreases.

Figure 13 - Algorithm for choosing statistical tests.

Test the normality of the distribution				Kolmogorov-Smirnov Test Shapiro-Wilk Test
Compare a variable between 2 or more groups				
Compare results of a categorical variable	Independent groups	2 groups	Binary variable	Fisher's Exact Test or Chi-Square Test
			Variable with more than 2 categories	Chi-Square Test
		More than 2 groups	Variable with more than 2 categories	Chi-Square Test
	Dependent or paired groups	2 groups	Dependent or paired groups	McNemar test
Compare results of a continuous variable	Independent groups	2 groups	Normal distribution	T-test for independent samples
			Normal distribution	Mann-Whitney U test
		More than 2 groups	Normal distribution	ANOVA
			Non-normal distribution	Kruskal-Wallis test
	Dependent or paired groups	2 groups	Normal distribution	T-test for dependent or paired samples
			Non-normal distribution	Wilcoxon test
		More than 2 groups	Normal distribution	Repeated Measures ANOVA
			Non-normal distribution	Friedman test
Testing the association between 2 variables				
Test the association between two continuous numerical variables			Normal distribution	Pearson's correlation
			Non-normal distribution	Spearman correlation
Testing the association between two ordinal variables				Spearman correlation
Testing the association between two categorical variables				Chi-Square Test

We say that a correlation is significant (positive or negative) depending on the sign of the r value and the associated p value.

If we want to analyze the association between categorical variables, we will actually proceed in the same way as in the comparison of a categorical variable between groups. In this case, you are not dealing with groups, but with some other variable also defined in the form of categories. For example, consider that you want to verify if there is an association between having a high level of knowledge about specific LGBTQIA+ health issues and sexual orientation. In this case, you would use a Chi-square test.

Practical Applications

Consider a study that aims to evaluate a new pain reliever, comparing it to a control treatment. We define the primary endpoint as the percentage of people without pain 2 hours after taking the drug.

In this case, we have:

- Objective: To compare the percentage of successes in the group of people who took drug A with the group of people who took the control.

- Number of groups: 2 independent groups (the results of people in the group who took drug A are not influenced by the results of people who took the control).

- Variable: Number of successes, categorical binary variable (success - no pain at 2h/failure - pain at 2h).

- Significance: 0.05

Results obtained in the sample studied: successes with drug A – 68%; successes with control – 56%

Let's follow the algorithm presented above to determine which tests to use:

1. Independent groups;

2. Comparison of a variable between 2 groups;

3. Binary variable;

4. Fisher's Exact Test or Chi-Square Test.

The statistical test to be considered is Fisher's exact test or, alternatively, the Chi-square test. The test is performed using statistical analysis software and, if the p-value associated with the test is less than 0.05 (less than the significance value defined for the study), you should consider the difference between drug A and the control as statistically significant. Otherwise, you would have to conclude that the difference in your sample was 12%, but when extrapolated to the population, this difference is not statistically significant. In other words, there is a probability greater than 5% that the difference found may be due to chance and not to a real difference between the drugs.

Let's look at another example, consider the same study, but now the endpoint defined for pain assessment is the percentage reduction in pain, evaluated by a VAS scale (0 to 10 points), 1 hour after administration of drug A or control. In other words, what we want to compare is the average percentage reduction in the group that took drug A versus the average percentage reduction in the group that took the control.

In this case, we have:

• Objective: to compare the percentage reduction in pain, assessed by a VAS scale (0 to 10 points), 1 hour after taking drug A or control.

• Number of groups: 2 independent groups.

• Variable: Mean percentage reduction in pain scale after 1 hour in each group; (baseline VAS - VAS after 1h)/(baseline VAS) x100.

• Significance: 0.05

Results obtained in the sample studied: mean reduction of drug A - 43%; standard deviation - 34%; mean reduction of control - 36%; standard deviation - 32%.

Let's follow the algorithm presented above:

1. Continuous numerical variable;

2. Independent groups;

3. Compare a variable between 2 groups;

4. If the variable has a normal distribution - T-test for independent samples; If the variable has a non-normal distribution - Mann-Whitney test.

The statistical test to be considered is the T-test for independent samples, if the variable has a normal distribution. If the variable mean percentage reduction in pain scale after 1 hour does not have a normal distribution, or if you assume that you do not know the type of distribution of the variable, you can opt for the so-called non-parametric tests, which do not assume a specific distribution of the data (i.e., they do not require a normal distribution). In this context, you can use the Mann-Whitney test as an alternative to the T-test for independent samples.

Other Statistical Analyses

There are numerous statistical analyses beyond those mentioned above, which are beyond the scope of this manual. However, I would like to mention a few that deserve to be highlighted, both for the type of analysis they use and for the frequency with which they are applied.

Survival analysis

In this type of analysis, the term survival is used, but it doesn't necessarily refer to literal survival, but rather the occurrence of a specific event. Survival analysis is a statistical method used to analyze the time until a certain event occurs. In formal terms, it assesses the probability of an event not occurring at a given time point.

Some of the most common techniques are Kaplan-Meier analysis and the Log-Rank test.

Kaplan-Meier analysis is a non-parametric method that estimates the survival function from observed data with censored values. During the analyzed period, some individuals may not experience the event of interest or may be lost to follow-up. Their data is considered censored and methods are used to account for this. Results are usually presented in the form of curves.

The Log-Rank test allows you to compare the survival curves of two or more groups to determine if there are significant differences.

Regression analysis

Regression analysis is a statistical method that evaluates whether there is a relationship between one variable, called the dependent variable, and other variables, called independent variables. There are different types of regression analysis, such as simple linear regression, multiple linear regression, and logistic regression.

Simple linear regression describes the relationship between two variables, allowing the prediction of one as a function of the other, assuming they are linearly related.

Multiple linear regression creates a model that explains a continuous numerical dependent variable as a function of several other variables.

Logistic regression is a technique that evaluates the association between a binary (or categorical) variable and a set of continuous or categorical variables. Results are presented in the form of odds ratios and their respective p-values.

Chapter 32 - Sample Size and Sample Characteristics

The vast majority of clinical studies are conducted based on a sample. In other words, a small group of people with certain characteristics (defined by inclusion and exclusion criteria) is studied and, based on the results obtained, the findings are estimated for the population as a whole. The population is understood here as all people with similar characteristics to the sample studied.

To have a representative sample, that is, capable of accurately predicting the results for the target population, two aspects must be taken into account: the number of people included in the sample and their diversity.

In the next pages, we will see how to determine the number of people to be included in a given study.

Regarding the diversity of people included, this is especially relevant in population-based epidemiological studies. In these studies, for example, to estimate the frequency of an event, such as the prevalence of a disease in a country or region, samples need not only to be of an adequate size, but must also reflect the national or regional diversity.

Consider, for example, a study to assess the prevalence of obesity in the New York City metropolitan area. Obviously, the first thing to do is determine the number of people to be included in the sample. As we will see next, this number depends on your objective, in this case, estimating a frequency, the frequency you expect to obtain, which is based on already published information, and the margin of error you consider for your estimate. Let's focus for now on the diversity of the sample. Regardless of the number of people you include, it will be necessary to ensure that they come from different zones of the area and that people of different genders and ages are included, according to the area's pattern, which can be defined, for example, from census data (which may mean that, due to lack of data, you will not be able to stratify the samples according to all the characteristics you would like).

Determining the sample size

Sample sizes can be calculated using specific statistical software (I suggest two of the many free software packages for sample size calculation: https://www.openepi.com/ and https://sample-size.net/).
However, whichever program is chosen, you will always have to define for yourself the premises on which the calculation is based. In this manual, we will discuss sample calculation in some common situations.

The first thing you need to do to determine the size of a sample is to define its significance (see chapter 29 for more information on significance) and, in the case of a comparative study, you also need to determine the study power (see chapter 29 for more information on study power).

Next, discuss the objective of the study. Different objectives imply different samples, and there is no magic number that is considered a representative or significant sample.

In a simplified way, we can divide studies into three types: studies that aim to determine a frequency, like the one we just saw about the prevalence of obesity, studies that aim to compare frequencies, and studies that aim to compare mean values. Survival estimates, median comparisons, or odds ratio estimates are outside the scope of this manual.

To calculate the sample needed for a study to determine the frequency of an event, the following must be taken into account:

- What is the size of the population to which the results should be extrapolated? However, it is considered that for large populations, above 100,000, the change to higher values has no impact on the calculation of the sample size.

- What is the expected frequency of the event (based on the literature or your own expectations).

- What sampling error do you accept (what will be the width of the confidence interval).

- The study's significance level.

In studies designed to compare frequencies, it is necessary to determine:

- What is the expected difference between the two groups to be compared or what is the expected frequency for each of the groups (based on the literature or your own expectations).

- The significance level and study power.

In studies designed to compare differences between means, it is necessary to determine:

- What is the expected difference between the means of the two groups and what is the standard deviation of the difference or the standard deviation and mean of each group (based on the literature or your own expectations).

- The significance level and study power.

Let's take a look at some practical examples. Consider a study whose objective is to determine the frequency of an event. When evaluating your sample, you will obtain a point estimate value and estimate the value for the population, which means that you will calculate the confidence interval (the range where the true frequency of the population will be).

Let's go back to the previous example, where we wanted to assess the prevalence of obesity in the New York City metropolitan area. Let's define the premises for calculating the sample:

Significance - 0.05 (that is, assuming 95% confidence intervals).

Estimated value for the prevalence of obesity - 22% (estimated from the literature).

Width of the confidence interval (sampling error) - 3% (empirically defined by the research team).

The sample consists of 732 people (https://www.openepi.com/).

But if, instead of a significance of 0.05, we assume a significance of 0.01 (99% confidence intervals), the sample value will be 1,264 people.

If, instead of a 3% confidence interval (which means that, if the value found in our study is 22%, we can say that the value for the New York City metropolitan population will be between 19% and 25%), we assume that we want to have a narrower interval, for example, 2% (which means that, if the value found in our study is 22%, we can say that the value for the New York City metropolitan population will be between 20% and 24%), the sample size will be 1,646 people for a 95% confidence interval and 2,839 for a 99% confidence interval.

In summary, the sample you need for this study will be as large as:

- If you use 99% confidence intervals instead of 95% (greater certainty in the estimate);

- The closer to 50% the estimated value of the event you are evaluating is;

- The smaller the width of the estimated interval.

Remember the study from the previous chapter that compared the success rate of the group of people taking drug A with the group of people taking the control for pain relief?

> Objective: Compare the success rate in the group of people taking drug A with the group of people taking the control.
>
> Number of groups: 2 independent groups.
>
> Variable: number of successes, categorical variable, binary (success - no pain at 2 hours/failure - pain at 2 hours).
>
> Significance: 0.05.

What sample size would you need for this study? Let's define the premises for calculating the sample:

> Significance - 0.05 (that is, assuming 95% confidence intervals).
>
> Study power - 90% (that is, you have a 90% probability of detecting the difference, if it exists).

Estimated difference between the groups - To make the calculation, it is necessary to determine what result (success) you expect (based on the literature and previous studies) for the control group and by how much you assume drug A will be different. Consider that previous results for the control point to a 50% success rate and that you want your study to detect a difference of at least 10%, if any.

The estimated sample size is 538 people in each group (https://sample-size.net/).

However, if instead of assuming 90% power, you assume 80% power, the estimated sample size would be 408 people per group. If you assume 80% power and a difference between groups of at least 15% rather than 10%, the estimated sample size would be 183 people per group.

Adjusting the Sample Size for Potential Dropouts

If you anticipate there may be dropouts during the study (participants who do not make it to the end), you need to account for this when calculating the sample size. You should assume an expected value for the dropout rate and recalculate the sample size with this in mind. For example, if for a given study it was calculated based on the applicable assumptions that 100 participants need to be included, and if a 10% dropout rate is expected, then the study should include 112 people. There is often the mistaken approach of estimating an additional 10% over the required sample size, which in this case would result in 110 people per group, but if you lose 10% from a group of 110 people, that equates to losing 11 people, which means that in the end you would have 99 people and not the required 100.

Bibliography

1. Constitution of the World Health Organization [Internet]. [cited 2023 Jun 12]. Available from: https://www.who.int/about/governance/constitution

2. Cavazzoni P, Anagnostiadis E, Ph R, Lolic M. 2020 Drug Trials Snapshots Summary Report. 2020;

3. Census Bureau Tables [Internet]. [cited 2023 Sep 20]. Available from: https://data.census.gov/table?t=Age+and+Sex:Older+Population:Race+and+Ethnicity

4. Diversity and Inclusion in Clinical Trials: Bioethical Perspective and Principles [Internet]. IFPMA. [cited 2023 Sep 20]. Available from: https://www.ifpma.org/publications/diversity-and-inclusion-in-clinical-trials-bioethical-perspective-and-principles/

5. NIMHD [Internet]. [cited 2022 Dec 13]. Diversity and Inclusion in Clinical Trials. Available from: https://nimhd.nih.gov/resources/understanding-health-disparities/diversity-and-inclusion-in-clinical-trials.html

6. Embracing Diversity: The Imperative for Inclusive Clinical Trials [Internet]. 2023 [cited 2023 Sep 20]. Available from:

https://postgraduateeducation.hms.harvard.edu/trends-medicine/embracing-diversity-imperative-inclusive-clinical-trials

7. Diversity and inclusion in clinical research [Internet]. [cited 2023 Sep 20]. Available from: https://www.abpi.org.uk/r-d-manufacturing/clinical-research/diversity-and-inclusion-in-clinical-research/

8. Research C for DE and. Enhancing the Diversity of Clinical Trial Populations — Eligibility Criteria, Enrollment Practices, and Trial Designs Guidance for Industry [Internet]. FDA; 2020 [cited 2023 Sep 20]. Available from: https://www.fda.gov/regulatory-information/search-fda-guidance-documents/enhancing-diversity-clinical-trial-populations-eligibility-criteria-enrollment-practices-and-trial

9. Commissioner O of the. Collection of Race and Ethnicity Data in Clinical Trials [Internet]. FDA; 2023 [cited 2023 Sep 20]. Available from: https://www.fda.gov/regulatory-information/search-fda-guidance-documents/collection-race-and-ethnicity-data-clinical-trials

10. Considerations for the Inclusion of Adolescent Patients in Adult Oncology Clinical Trials, Guidance for Industry. Clinical Trials.

11. Minimum Age Considerations for Inclusion of Pediatric Patients [Internet]. [cited 2023 Sep 20]. Available from: https://www.fda.gov/media/121318/download

12. UNITED NATIONS Gender-inclusive language [Internet]. United Nations; [cited 2024 Feb 4]. Available from: https://www.un.org/en/gender-inclusive-language/guidelines.shtml

13. Identidade de género e orientação sexual na prática clínica. 1ª. Lisboa: Silabo; 2018. 185 p.

14. Fuentes A, Ackermann RR, Athreya S, Bolnick D, Lasisi T, Lee S, et al. AAPA Statement on Race and Racism. American J Phys Anthropol. 2019 Jul;169(3):400–2.

15. ICHGCP [Internet]. [cited 2022 Nov 21]. 1. GLOSSARY. Available from: https://ichgcp.net/1-glossary

16. Commissioner O of the. FDA. FDA; 2023 [cited 2024 Feb 4]. Real-World Evidence. Available from: https://www.fda.gov/science-research/science-and-research-special-topics/real-world-evidence

17. real-world-evidence-framework-support-eu-regulatory-decision-making-report-experience-gained_en.pdf [Internet]. [cited 2024 Feb 4]. Available from: https://www.ema.europa.eu/system/files/documents/report/real-world-evidence-framework-support-eu-regulatory-decision-making-report-experience-gained_en.pdf

18. WMA - The World Medical Association-WMA Declaration of Helsinki – Ethical Principles for Medical Research Involving Human Subjects [Internet]. [cited 2024 Feb 4]. Available from: https://www.wma.net/policies-post/wma-declaration-of-helsinki-ethical-principles-for-medical-research-involving-human-subjects/

19. Home | ClinicalTrials.gov [Internet]. [cited 2024 Feb 4]. Available from: https://clinicaltrials.gov/

20. Ratan SK, Anand T, Ratan J. Formulation of Research Question – Stepwise Approach. J Indian Assoc Pediatr Surg. 2019;24(1):15–20.

21. Brown D. A Review of the PubMed PICO Tool: Using Evidence-Based Practice in Health Education. Health Promot Pract. 2020 Jul;21(4):496–8.

22. Rios LP, Ye C, Thabane L. Association between framing of the research question using the PICOT format and reporting quality of randomized controlled trials. BMC Med Res Methodol. 2010 Feb 5;10:11.

23. Elias BL, Polancich S, Jones C, Convoy S. Evolving the PICOT Method for the Digital Age: The PICOT-D. J Nurs Educ. 2015 Oct;54(10):594–9.

24. Davies K. Formulating the Evidence Based Practice question: A review of the frameworks for LIS professionals. Evidence Based Library and Information Practice. 2011 Jun 24;6:75–80.

25. The research question in clinical practice: A guideline for its formulation [Internet]. [cited 2022 Nov 21]. Available from:

https://www.elsevier.es/en-revista-revista-colombiana-psiquiatria-english-edition--479-pdf-S2530312018300298

26. Aronson JK. Biomarkers and surrogate endpoints. Br J Clin Pharmacol. 2005 May;59(5):491–4.

27. Duffy SW, Treasure FP. Potential surrogate endpoints in cancer research--some considerations and examples. Pharm Stat. 2011 Feb;10(1):34–9.

28. Research C for DE and. Table of Surrogate Endpoints That Were the Basis of Drug Approval or Licensure. FDA [Internet]. 2022 Feb 28 [cited 2022 Nov 22]; Available from: https://www.fda.gov/drugs/development-resources/table-surrogate-endpoints-were-basis-drug-approval-or-licensure

29. Research C for DE and. Surrogate Endpoint Resources for Drug and Biologic Development. FDA [Internet]. 2021 Jan 29 [cited 2022 Nov 22]; Available from: https://www.fda.gov/drugs/development-resources/surrogate-endpoint-resources-drug-and-biologic-development

30. EQ-5D User Guides – EQ-5D [Internet]. [cited 2023 Jan 3]. Available from: https://euroqol.org/publications/user-guides/

31. GUIDELINE FOR GOOD CLINICAL PRACTICE.

32. Iasonos A, O'Quigley J. Design considerations for dose-expansion cohorts in phase I trials. J Clin Oncol. 2013 Nov 1;31(31):4014–21.

33. Boonstra PS, Braun TM, Chase EC. A modular framework for early-phase seamless oncology trials. Clin Trials. 2021 Jun;18(3):303–13.

34. Torres-Saavedra PA, Winter KA. An Overview of Phase 2 Clinical Trial Designs. International Journal of Radiation Oncology, Biology, Physics. 2022 Jan 1;112(1):22–9.

35. Commissioner O of the. Step 3: Clinical Research. FDA [Internet]. 2019 Apr 18 [cited 2022 Nov 22]; Available from: https://www.fda.gov/patients/drug-development-process/step-3-clinical-research

36. Ivy SP, Siu LL, Garrett-Mayer E, Rubinstein L. Approaches to phase 1 clinical trial design focused on safety, efficiency, and selected patient populations: a report from the clinical trial design task force of the national cancer institute investigational drug steering committee. Clin Cancer Res. 2010 Mar 15;16(6):1726–36.

37. van Gerven J, Cohen A. Integrating data from the Investigational Medicinal Product Dossier/investigator's brochure. A new tool for translational integration of preclinical effects. Br J Clin Pharmacol. 2018 Jul;84(7):1457–66.

38. Yan F, Thall PF, Lu KH, Gilbert MR, Yuan Y. Phase I–II clinical trial design: a state-of-the-art paradigm for dose finding. Ann Oncol. 2018 Mar;29(3):694–9.

39. Chilet-Rosell E. Gender bias in clinical research, pharmaceutical marketing, and the prescription of drugs. Glob Health Action. 2014;7:25484.

40. Liu KA, Mager NAD. Women's involvement in clinical trials: historical perspective and future implications. Pharm Pract (Granada). 2016;14(1):708.

41. Zakhem GA, Motosko CC, Mu EW, Ho RS. Infertility and teratogenicity after paternal exposure to systemic dermatologic medications: A systematic review. J Am Acad Dermatol. 2019 Apr;80(4):957–69.

42. Lutwak-Mann C, Schmid K, Keberle H. Thalidomide in Rabbit Semen. Nature. 1967 Jun;214(5092):1018–20.

43. Prout MN, Fish SS. Participation of women in clinical trials of drug therapies: a context for the controversies. Medscape Womens Health. 2001 Oct;6(5):1.

44. U.S. Food and Drug Administration. Guideline for the study and evaluation of gender differences in the clinical evaluation of drugs; notice. Fed Regist. 1993 Jul 22;58(139):39406–16.

45. Pinnow E, Sharma P, Parekh A, Gevorkian N, Uhl K. Increasing participation of women in early phase clinical trials approved by the FDA. Womens Health Issues. 2009 Apr;19(2):89–93.

46. Chilet-Rosell E, Ruiz-Cantero MT, Horga JF. Women's health and gender-based clinical trials on etoricoxib: methodological gender bias. J Public Health (Oxf). 2009 Sep;31(3):434–45.

47. Ruiz-Cantero MT, Blasco-Blasco M, Chilet-Rosell E, Peiró AM. Gender bias in therapeutic effort: from research to health care. Farm Hosp. 2020 Apr 14;44(3):109–13.

48. Yang Y, Carlin AS, Faustino PJ, Motta MIP, Hamad ML, He R, et al. Participation of women in clinical trials for new drugs approved by the food and drug administration in 2000-2002. J Womens Health (Larchmt). 2009 Mar;18(3):303–10.

49. Merck Sharp & Dohme LLC. A Phase 1, Open-Label, Non-Randomized, 2-Period, Fixed Sequence, Study to Assess the Absolute Bioavailability and Fraction Absorbed of Ertugliflozin in Health Male Subjects Using a 14^C-Microdose Approach [Internet]. clinicaltrials.gov; 2018 Aug [cited 2022 Nov 21]. Report No.: NCT02411929. Available from: https://clinicaltrials.gov/ct2/show/NCT02411929

50. MacroGenics. A Phase 1 Study to Evaluate the Safety, Immunologic and Virologic Responses of MGD014 Therapy in HIV-Infected Individuals on Suppressive Antiretroviral Therapy [Internet]. clinicaltrials.gov; 2022 Aug [cited 2022 Nov 21]. Report No.: NCT03570918. Available from: https://clinicaltrials.gov/ct2/show/NCT03570918

51. Renfro LA, Sargent DJ. Statistical controversies in clinical research: basket trials, umbrella trials, and other master protocols: a review and examples. Ann Oncol. 2017 Jan 1;28(1):34–43.

52. Park JJH, Hsu G, Siden EG, Thorlund K, Mills EJ. An overview of precision oncology basket and umbrella trials for clinicians. CA: A Cancer Journal for Clinicians. 2020;70(2):125–37.

53. Parmar MK, Sydes MR, Cafferty FH, Choodari-Oskooei B, Langley RE, Brown L, et al. Testing many treatments within a single protocol over 10 years at MRC CTU at UCL: Multi-arm, multi stage platform, umbrella and basket protocols. Clin Trials. 2017 Oct;14(5):451–61.

54. Idera Pharmaceuticals, Inc. A Phase 1/2 Study to Assess the Safety and Efficacy of Intratumoral IMO-2125 in Combination With Ipilimumab or Pembrolizumab in Patients With Metastatic Melanoma (ILLUMINATE-204) [Internet]. clinicaltrials.gov; 2022 Jul [cited 2022 Dec 2]. Report No.: NCT02644967. Available from: https://clinicaltrials.gov/ct2/show/NCT02644967

55. Calithera Biosciences, Inc. A Multicenter Phase 2 Study of the Glutaminase Inhibitor CB-839 in Combination With Paclitaxel in Patients With Advanced Triple Negative Breast Cancer (TNBC) Including Patients of African Ancestry and Non-African Ancestry [Internet]. clinicaltrials.gov; 2022 Sep [cited 2024 Jan 1]. Report No.: NCT03057600. Available from: https://clinicaltrials.gov/study/NCT03057600

56. Cipriani A, Barbui C. What is a factorial trial? Epidemiol Psychiatr Sci. 2013 May 16;22(3):213–5.

57. NOT-OD-18-014: Revision: NIH Policy and Guidelines on the Inclusion of Women and Minorities as Subjects in Clinical Research [Internet]. [cited 2022 Dec 13]. Available from: https://grants.nih.gov/grants/guide/notice-files/NOT-OD-18-014.html

58. Geller SE, Koch AR, Roesch P, Filut A, Hallgren E, Carnes M. The More Things Change, the More They Stay the Same: A Study to Evaluate Compliance With Inclusion and Assessment of Women and Minorities in Randomized Controlled Trials. Acad Med. 2018 Apr;93(4):630–5.

59. Khan MS, Shahid I, Siddiqi TJ, Khan SU, Warraich HJ, Greene SJ, et al. Ten-Year Trends in Enrollment of Women and Minorities in Pivotal Trials Supporting Recent US Food and Drug Administration Approval of Novel Cardiometabolic Drugs. J Am Heart Assoc. 2020 Jun 13;9(11):e015594.

60. Commissioner O of the. U.S. Food and Drug Administration. FDA; 2022 [cited 2022 Dec 13]. Diversity Plans to Improve Enrollment of Participants From Underrepresented Racial and Ethnic Populations in Clinical Trials; Draft Guidance for Industry; Availability. Available from: https://www.fda.gov/regulatory-information/search-fda-guidance-documents/diversity-plans-improve-enrollment-participants-underrepresented-racial-and-ethnic-populations

61. Hwang TJ, Brawley OW. New Federal Incentives for Diversity in Clinical Trials. New England Journal of Medicine. 2022 Oct 13;387(15):1347–9.

62. Loree JM, Anand S, Dasari A, Unger JM, Gothwal A, Ellis LM, et al. Disparity of Race Reporting and Representation in Clinical Trials Leading to Cancer Drug Approvals From 2008 to 2018. JAMA Oncology. 2019 Oct 10;5(10):e191870.

63. Rosenson RS. Comparative Efficacy of Ticagrelor Versus Aspirin on Blood Viscosity in Peripheral Artery Disease Patients with Type 2 Diabetes. 2015;(2).

64. GlaxoSmithKline. A Multicenter, Randomized, Double-Blind, Parallel Group, 52-Week Comparison of Asthma Control and Measures of Airway Inflammation in Subjects of African Descent Receiving Fluticasone Propionate/Salmeterol 100/50mcg DISKUS® BID or Fluticasone Propionate 100mcg DISKUS® BID Alone [Internet]. clinicaltrials.gov; 2017 Jan [cited 2024 Jan 1]. Report No.: NCT00102765. Available from: https://clinicaltrials.gov/study/NCT00102765

65. Kamen C. Exercise Intervention for Lesbian, Gay, Bisexual, and Transgender (LGBT) Cancer Survivors and Caregivers [Internet]. clinicaltrials.gov; 2023 Feb [cited 2024 Jan 1]. Report No.: NCT02459769. Available from: https://clinicaltrials.gov/study/NCT02459769

66. Jones H. Stress-reduction Wellness Program for Midlife Black Women (B-SWELL) [Internet]. clinicaltrials.gov; 2023 Jan [cited 2024 Jan 1]. Report No.: NCT04404478. Available from: https://clinicaltrials.gov/study/NCT04404478

67. Macedo A, Aurindo M, Febra C. Effectiveness of undergraduate medical students training on LGBTQIA+ people health: a systematic review and meta-analysis. BMC Med Educ. 2024 Jan 16;24(1):63.

68. Agénor M, Pérez AE, Tabaac AR, Bond KT, Charlton BM, Bowen DJ, et al. Sexual Orientation Identity Disparities in Mammography Among White, Black, and Latina U.S. Women. LGBT Health. 2020 Jul 13;7(6):312–20.

69. Cochran SD, Mays VM. Risk of breast cancer mortality among women cohabiting with same sex partners: findings from the National Health Interview Survey, 1997-2003. J Womens Health (Larchmt). 2012 May;21(5):528–33.

70. Framingham Heart Study [Internet]. [cited 2024 Feb 28]. Available from: https://www.framinghamheartstudy.org/

71. Gorbach P. Transmission Behavior in Partnerships of Newly HIV Infected Southern Californians [Internet]. clinicaltrials.gov; 2019 Apr [cited 2024 Jan 1]. Report No.: NCT01201083. Available from: https://clinicaltrials.gov/study/NCT01201083

72. Men Who Have Sex with Men (MSM) [Internet]. 2022 [cited 2024 Feb 3]. Available from: https://www.cdc.gov/std/treatment-guidelines/msm.htm

73. Ishikane M, Arima Y, Itoda I, Yamagishi T, Takahashi T, Matsui T, et al. Case-control study of risk factors for incident syphilis infection among men who have sex with men in Tokyo, Japan. Western Pac Surveill Response J. 2019 Dec 9;10(4):1–8.

74. National Cancer Institute (NCI). Case-Control Study of Renal Cell Cancer Among Caucasians and African Americans in the United States [Internet]. clinicaltrials.gov; 2020 Dec [cited 2024 Jan 1]. Report No.: NCT00340457. Available from: https://clinicaltrials.gov/study/NCT00340457

75. Van Wagoner NJ, Harbison HS, Drewry J, Turnipseed E, Hook EW. Characteristics of Women Reporting Multiple Recent Sex Partners Presenting to a Sexually Transmitted Disease Clinic for Care. Sexually Transmitted Diseases. 2011 Mar;38(3):210–5.

76. Muzny DC. A Case Control Study of Women With Multiple Sexual Partners Attending the Jefferson County Department of Health Sexually Transmitted Diseases Clinic [Internet]. clinicaltrials.gov; 2017 May [cited 2024 Jan 1]. Report No.: NCT01578915. Available from: https://clinicaltrials.gov/study/NCT01578915

77. Severo M, Santos AC, Lopes C, Barros H. [Reliability and validity in measuring physical and mental health construct of the Portuguese version of MOS SF-36]. Acta Med Port. 2006;19(4):281–7.

About the Author

Ana Macedo, 51 years old, 5 children, physician, graduated in 1997 from the University of Lisbon School of Medicine. PhD in Pharmacology from the Autonomous University of Barcelona. Academic title of aggregation from the University of the Algarve.

Currently she is an Invited Associate Professor with Aggregation at the Faculty of Medicine and Biomedical Sciences at the University of Algarve. Director of the PhD Program in Clinical Research and Translational Medicine at the University of Algarve. Chair of the Ethics Committee of the Algarve Biomedical Center.

Author of the books, Como Nascem Novos Medicamentos', 'Estatística Precisa-se'. 'A Saúde não ter Preço mas tem Custos', e 'Identidade de Género e Orientação Sexual na Prática Clínica'.

www.ingramcontent.com/pod-product-compliance
Lightning Source LLC
Chambersburg PA
CBHW050204230526
45470CB00001B/237